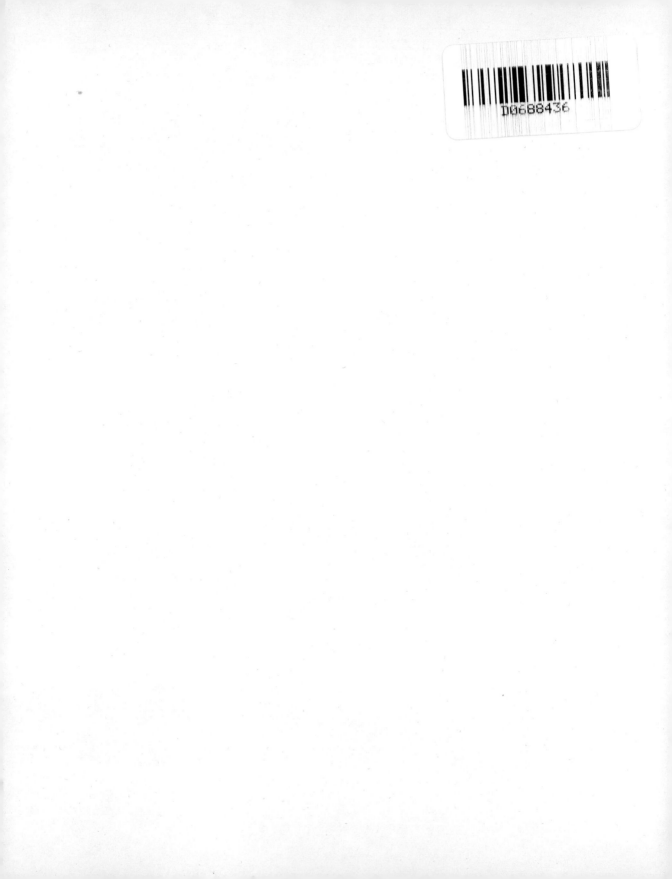

D0688436

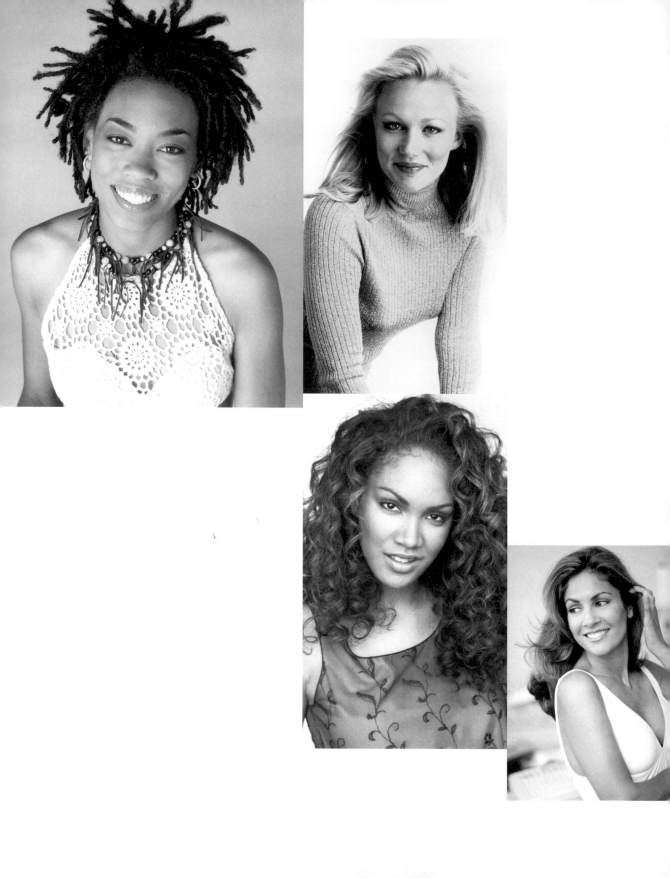

andretalkshair!

With a Special Message from OPRAH WINFREY

ANDRE WALKER with Teresa Wiltz

SIMON & SCHUSTER

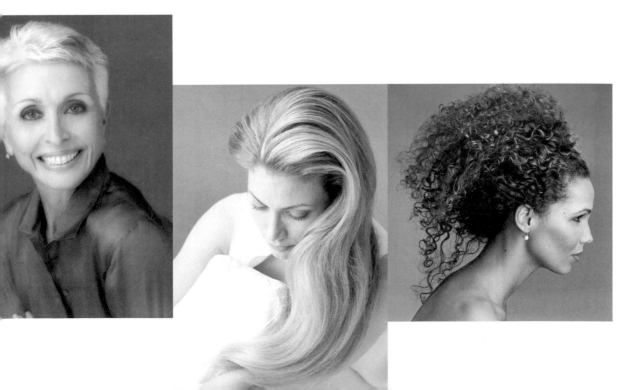

SIMON & SCHUSTER

Rockefeller Center

1230 Avenue of the Americas

New York, NY 10020

Copyright © 1997 by Andre Walker

All rights reserved,

including the right of reproduction

in whole or in part in any form.

SIMON & SCHUSTER and colophon are registered trademarks

of Simon & Schuster Inc.

Designed by Bonni Leon-Berman

Creative direction by Cynthia Moore

Photographed by John Beckett

with contributing photographs by Darcy McGrath

Manufactured in the United States of America

10 9 8 7 6 5 4 3 2 1

Library of Congress Cataloging-in-Publication Data

Walker, Andre.

Andre talks hair! / Andre Walker with Teresa Wiltz ;

with a special message from Oprah Winfrey.

p. cm.

Includes index.

1. Hairdressing. 2. Hair—Care and hygiene. I. Wiltz, Teresa.

II. Title.

TT972.W25   1997

646.7'24—dc21   97-3510 CIP

ISBN 0-684-82456-6

contents

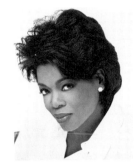

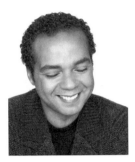

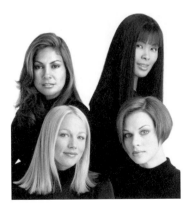

contents

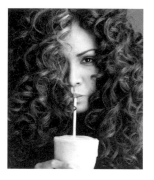
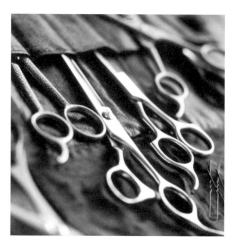
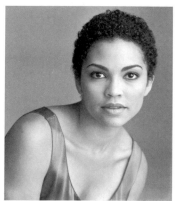

contents

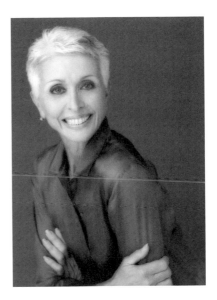

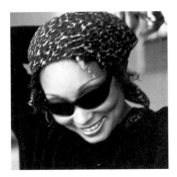

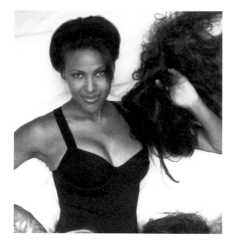

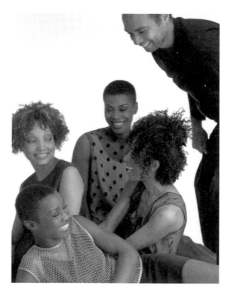

contents

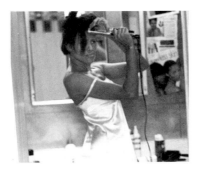

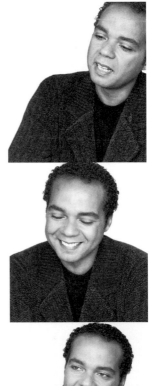

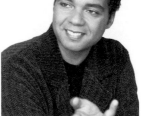

foreword by **oprah winfrey**

could talk for hours about hair and how much it meant to me while growing up with my grandmother in rural Kosciusko, Mississippi. Back then, hair played a prominent part in my life. Every day, my grandmother used to sit me down and give me three fat plaits—two sticking from the back of my head and another one twisted in the front. On holidays and special occasions, I got to wear my hair down in much–wished for and admired Shirley Temple curls, with one big roll in the front for bangs—because my grandmother, Hattie Mae, didn't want to cut my hair, not even enough for bangs. One thing I knew for sure was that my hair was very thick. Sisters in the church, relatives and even folks who barely knew me were always telling me, "Ooooh, that child has a lot of hair," they used to say. "What's Hattie Mae goin' do with all that child's thick hair? It's a lot to keep up."

It *was* a lot to keep up. Still, some of my most comforting memories are of sitting between my grandmother's skirted knees while she scratched my head and oiled my scalp. It was our ritual, one we performed again and again, right there on the front porch—as did many a black girl growing up in the South. Today, I know enough to know that comfort was about all that I was getting out of our little ritual, because it certainly wasn't doing my hair a bit of good. But it felt great at the time. We were told on many a day, "Child, your hair is your crowning glory." We risked the wrath of the ancestors—or worse, the living—if we dared cut it. Needless to say, I didn't cut mine for years, except maybe to trim the ends. Hair was to be revered, admired.

That's true even today, no matter what your race or where you're from. Like it or not, we are a society that makes judgments about people based on what they look like. And hair is a big part of how you look. I wish it weren't that way, but that's the way it is. Hair is one of the defining statements about your style, of who you are and what you present to the world. When your hair is clean, shiny and cared for, people take notice. You can have the finest dress on, the best shoes, all the greatest accessories, Cartier to the bone—if your hair is not in order, it doesn't matter.

But it's how you feel about your own hair that matters more than anything. Hair grows on your head; your attitude about it grows *in* your head. We all have a certain image of how we want to look. We want to use all that we have to its greatest potential. It's hard to do that if you feel like your hair isn't looking its best. When my hair is looking bad, I don't feel good about myself. Other people might say I look terrific, but if *I* don't think I look terrific, then I don't.

And trust me, there have been lots of times when my hair didn't look so good. I don't think there's a woman out there who doesn't have at least one hair nightmare to talk about. I've had more than my share.

Once, when I was just starting out in television news, I went to one of those fancy salons in New York City. I knew enough about the difference between Caucasian hair and black women's hair to at least ask the fancy salon owner, who was French, if they did black hair. He said, *"Oui, Madam,* we do black hair, we do red hair, we do blond hair, we do your hair." I was twenty-two and didn't have the kind of courage then that I've since grown into. So when this Frenchman put a "French" perm into my non-French hair, I let him. He went off to attend to some other redhead, blonde or brunette while I sat there, letting the perm burn into my cerebral cortex. When he finally came back to check on me, I said, "I think this needs to come off now. It's really burning." He looked at the container and said, "No, you need at least eight more minutes." By this time, my eyes were tearing and I could feel scabs forming on my head. When he finally rinsed the perm out, my whole head was one big scab holding in the hair follicles. I went home, my head throbbing.

In a week, half of all my hair had fallen out. Every time I combed it, I would get another handful of hair. I walked around with bald patches in my hair for at least a week, until a friend in the newsroom pulled me aside and said, "I know you're trying to hold onto your hair, but you really don't have any. You're looking bad, sister. Why don't you come and go with me to my barber and we can shave your head." I went home and cried and then took a good look at myself in the mirror. She was right.

So the next day, I went to the barber and had my head shaved. Horror of horrors. I couldn't find a wig to fit my bald head—my head is twenty-five and a quarter inches round. (When I did the movie *The Color Purple,* the hairdressers had to sew two wigs together to fit my head.) So there I was, an anchorwoman on television with a shaved head. I couldn't even figure out how to tie scarves just right to hide my baldness. Finally, little pieces of fuzz started to grow back. After that, I was so afraid of any chemicals that I did not go to a beauty salon for six straight years—I wore a 'fro. Friends would say, "Don't you know that 'fros are 'out'?" My response? "This is the only way I'm going to wear my hair." I was afraid to trust any hairdressers.

Finally, just before I moved to Chicago to do *The Oprah Winfrey Show,* I tried lightly perming my hair for a Jheri curl–style 'do—without the grease. Unfortunately, the hairdresser who put in the light perm didn't wash it all out in the back. So my hair started to fall out in patches. Again. And once again, I shaved my head down to a little teeny weeny Afro. I was batting zero with hairdressers.

Until I met Andre. One day, I was out shopping and noticed an attractive black woman with hair that appeared to be the same texture as mine, but her hair had shine and movement and was obviously very healthy. I asked her, "How'd you get hair like that?" She told me about her hairdresser, Andre Walker. By coincidence, Andre had recently sent me flowers, trying to convince me to let him do my hair. So I invited him to the studio for a tryout. After all my experiences, I was reluctant to trust him. The first time he did my hair, it looked really great. But how was I to know that it wasn't going to fall out the next day? It didn't fall out, so I called him back for another tryout. I called him again, and again and again. I grew to trust him. For more than eleven years, Andre has been the man, the *only* man, who handles my hair.

The thing about Andre that I really appreciate is that he understands hair *and* he loves it. He loves what hair does, he loves its texture, he loves to play with it. Whenever you find someone who loves their work, they're usually better at it than anyone else. The industry apparently agrees with me; he's won five Emmys for doing my hair.

Those Emmys are well deserved. My hair has become stronger, healthier. Andre understands my hair and keeps me looking current without mimicking other people's hairdos. I've evolved and so has my hair; my hair has seen different lengths and different moods. I've always made a conscious effort to not get stuck in life—to keep growing, getting better and getting stronger. That's exactly what should happen to you and your hair. Many women get stuck in one look. But hair grows and you can always change it. A hairstyle is the easiest thing to change, for goodness sake.

Hair should be fun. Hair should move, and it should be friendly. Hair should be an invitation; people should look at it and want to touch it. We all need to strike a balance in life between trying new things and finding what's best for us. Don't take yourself—or your hair—too seriously.

Which is why you've got Andre—and this book. With Andre's help, you'll come away understanding your own hair, your hair type, what to expect from your hair, its possibilities. Like me, you can develop a greater and more realistic expectation for what your particular hair type can and absolutely cannot do. You don't have to walk around trying to have Diana Ross or Cindy Crawford hair. Andre can help you make your hair be its best in terms of strength, vitality, beauty, shine—all that good stuff.

What more can I say? I don't know where my hair would be without Andre. He's helped me to take care of it; with him, I've learned to love it, too. And in eleven years, I haven't had to shave my head once.

andretalkshair...

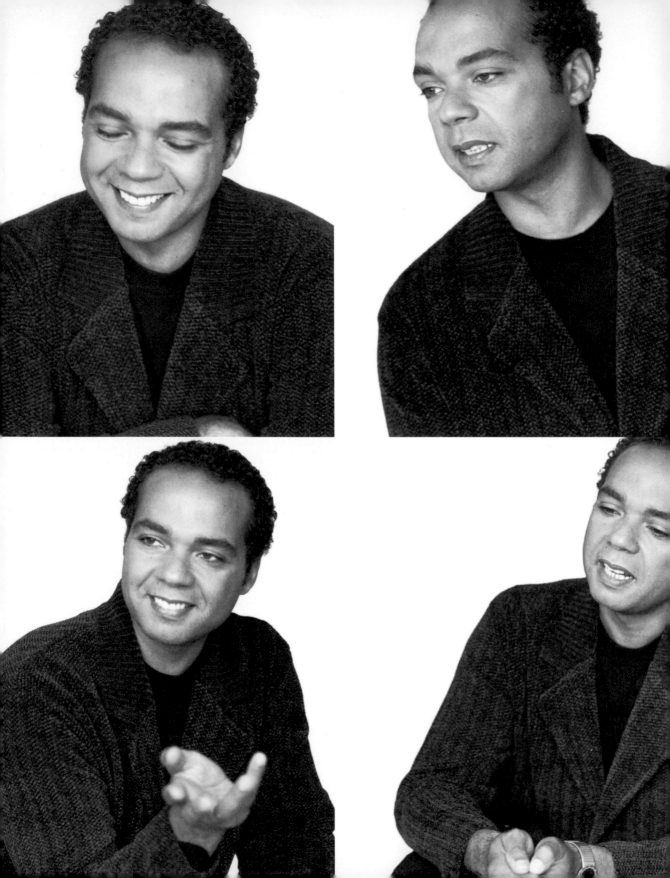

getting
to know
me

Let's face it: When it comes to hair, few women are content with the beauty God handed out at birth. Even if she's a modern-day Rapunzel, the average woman will find some little something she'd love to change about her hair. So what does she do? She fries it, dyes it, perms it, irons it, conks it, curls it, relaxes it, sprays it, frizzes it, sticks it with pins, hacks it off, stretches it with extensions or beats it with a blow-dryer. Then, when it's breaking off in clumps, she runs to a hairdresser or dashes to a drugstore in search of that magic elixir to erase all the horrors she's just inflicted upon her tresses.

Some of this dissatisfaction is a simple grass-is-always-greener scenario. Some of it is good old cultural brainwashing: blondes have more fun. You won't be happy if you're nappy. Goldilocks. The Breck Girl. Those glossy magazine photos of glamorous supermodels with long, flowing locks—never mind that it took an army of hairstylists, photographers, styling products and a wind machine to achieve that "natural" look.

Enough is enough.

It's time for an attitude adjustment.

It's time for you to call a truce with your hair.

And I'm going to help you do it.

For the past decade, I've been working with Oprah Winfrey to achieve the dozens of hairstyles she's sported on and off the show. It may sound like I'm tooting my own horn, but Oprah's hair is enormously flattering—up-to-date yet classic, chic yet sassy, easy to care for, functional and, above all, healthy. Why? Because she works with what she's got, she isn't afraid to experiment *and* she follows my advice. By the end of this book, you'll be able to do the same—no matter what your race or hair type, no matter what monstrous acts you've committed on your hair.

Over the years, I've had the privilege of working with women in all walks of life, from celebrities like Halle Berry, Barbara Bush and Roseanne Barr to professional working women to my mother and sister. That's right, my mother and sister. They were my first clients—and very gracious guinea pigs, I might add. To this day, they won't let anyone else touch their hair.

You see, although I've been in the beauty business for more than twenty years, I've been fascinated with hair since I was a little kid growing up in Chicago. By the time I was in junior high, I decided that I could style hair. And so I did, messing with my sister Pam's hair every chance I got. Soon I was experimenting with my mother's wigs and wiglets. (Maybe I should have tried them first before I started going at my sister's hair!) It was fun, but I was just playing.

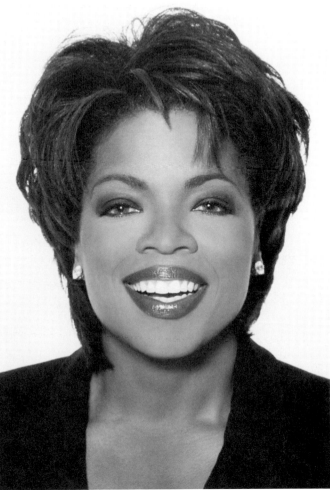

Skrebneski, © 1996, Harpo Productions, Inc.

Styling hair wasn't something that I took seriously until high school, when I won a hairstyling competition. The prize: a partial scholarship to Pivot Point Beauty College. I was thrilled—and so was Pam, who was my model. I accepted the scholarship, going to beauty school part-time until I graduated from high school. Then I made a decision that changed my life and freaked out my parents: I decided not to go to college. I knew the creative life of a hairstylist was the only life for me.

I was right. My career progressed rapidly as I worked in the best salons Chicago had to offer. By the time I was twenty-six, I had my own salon, naming it—

what else?—Andre Walker. Then Oprah moved to Chicago and my life changed. Again.

Through the grapevine, I heard that Oprah was looking for a stylist. I couldn't agree with her more. I saw how her hair looked on television, and I knew that I could make her look better. Much better. And that's exactly what I told her. Fortunately, she believed me. Now, like my mother and sister, she won't let anyone else touch her hair. The busier she is, the busier I am. My schedule is too hectic to accommodate running a business, but whenever I can, I squeeze in a couple of hours at a downtown salon in Chicago. Why? I like to make people look and *feel* good. Being able to dress hair isn't just being creative. It sounds hokey, but I really believe that helping other people feel better about themselves is my purpose in life.

Of course, we all know that looking good on the outside isn't going to help if you feel rotten on the inside. But looking good gives us all a little boost—not to mention the pleasure it gives the folks who have to look at us. What better way to attract attention than with a beautiful head of hair? Great hair is sensuous, pleasing to the eye and to the touch. We all want it. But beautiful hair shouldn't be your life's work. Find the easiest style for your hair to handle within its natural texture—and then forget about it. Until, of course, the compliments come pouring in.

Now, don't get me wrong. I'm not saying that you should never dye, relax or perm your hair. There's nothing wrong with a little artificial enhancement—I'm not against reaching for the chemicals or for a plug of synthetic hair. What's wrong is the spirit with which it is often done. This isn't war. Your hair isn't your enemy. It doesn't matter if you keep your hair natural or if you enhance the beauty God gave you. Whatever you do, it should be done in a playful spirit. Hair shouldn't have to be politically correct, but it shouldn't require a time-consuming, Herculean effort either.

Your hair *should* be easy to handle. You should love what you've got, whether it's bleached or jet black, straightened or kinky, wavy or stick straight, bouncin' and behavin' or limp and lank. All you need is a formula to make you look like a million bucks. And that's what I'm here for.

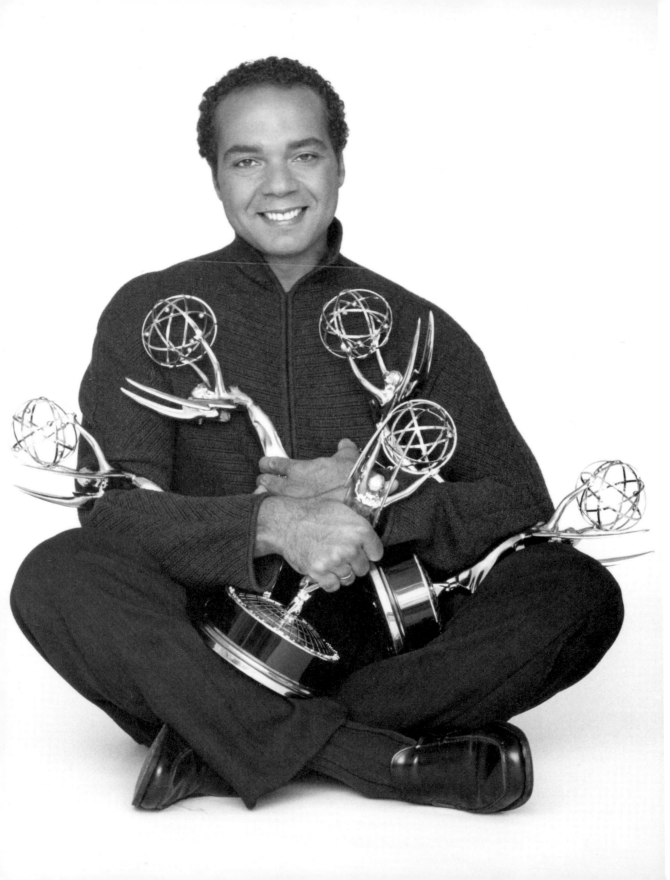

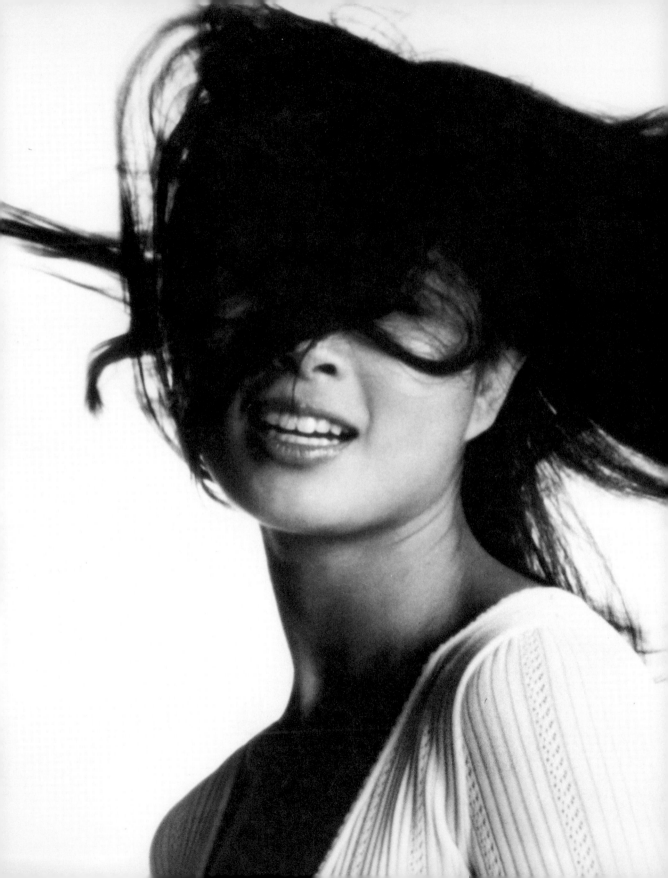

to thine
own self
be true

what's your type?

I've seen it happen time and time again. You know what I'm talking about. The "I-can't-do-a-thing-with-my-hair-so-now-I'm-really-going-to-screw-it-up" blues.

Maybe you've spent hundreds of dollars chasing that magic elixir guaranteed to give you, once and for all, hair that does exactly what you command it to do. You dash to the drugstore, where you find the perfect shampoo/conditioner/mousse/gel promised to fight frizz/create curl/boost body/thicken tresses/saturate shine. You ladle the goop onto your hair, comb it through, wait the prescribed five to thirty minutes and cross your fingers, hoping for a miracle. Only your hair looks exactly the same. Or even worse, it looks worse.

Or maybe, determined to give yourself a makeover, you've pored over page after page of those beauty magazines, analyzed your hair type, picked the perfect 'do and followed the directions step by step. Except that the directions could have been written in Sanskrit for all your hair cared. No matter how hard you try, your hair refuses to look like the model's in the photo. But it does look just like your toy poodle's.

Or maybe you've let someone talk you into getting that hot new perm/relaxer/hair-coloring technique. Until your hair grows out, you console yourself by sporting the latest look in crew cuts.

Or maybe your hair looks just great . . . as long as your hairstylist can squeeze you in at noon every Saturday. But whenever your stylist takes a vacation, so does your hair. Because in the privacy of your own bathroom, armed with a blow-dryer, you're all thumbs. Or perhaps you've found something that works just fine, but you always look the same and, well, you're bored.

Stop!

Your hair is not your enemy. It is not a rebellious child that must be wrestled into submission. It need not be a war.

No matter what the hair gurus out there may tell you, there is nothing mysterious about hair. It's a fabric, plain and simple. And just like other fabrics, there is no universal, one-size-fits-all approach for its care. You take care of a silk blouse differently from the way you do a cashmere sweater. Both are equally fabulous looking; both demand different formulas to keep them looking great. The same holds true for hair.

Think about it. If you had a formula to care for your mane, you'd bypass 95 percent of those magic elixirs. You'd think five times before consenting to a chemical process that might end up giving you a free haircut. You'd know how to help your hair look great all the time—even when your stylist is drinking daiquiris in Barbados.

But to get to that point, I want you to forget the old tried-and-not-so-true hair tales. Stop reading fashion magazines that tell you there's just one hair type if you're African-American, Asian, or whatever. Forget about race—there's no such thing as "black" hair or "Asian" hair or even "Caucasian" hair. And, please, please, please, let's retire forever those antiquated stereotypes about "good" hair versus "bad" hair.

The fact is, everyone has "good" hair—you just have to know how to take care of your hair type. Obviously, folks from certain ethnic groups are more likely to fit more into one category than another. But

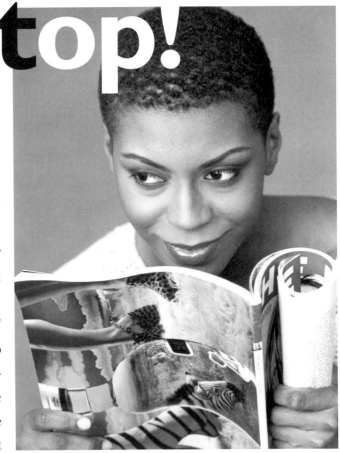

what if your hair doesn't fit into the predefined category for your race? You can be African-American with naturally stick-straight hair, or you can be a kinky-haired Irish-American. And because our country is becoming such a multiracial hybrid, it just doesn't make sense anymore to stick to such rigid definitions. It's time to throw out the rule books. It's time for a new approach. It's time to get rid of the grass-is-always-greener mentality. We always want what we don't have. I'd like to see women really appreciate what they do have and make it work for them.

Believe me, making your hair work for you isn't that hard. You just need an expert to guide you, and here I am. During my twenty years in the business dealing with every kind of hair known to woman, I've found that there are just four distinct hair types. Within those hair types, there may be variations on a theme—let's call them subtypes. If you know and understand your true hair type, you'll be able to find a formula that will let you take care of your mane with ease. Even if you're dead set on working against Mother Nature, you won't have to do major battle to make your hair do what you want it to.

But before I tell you my secrets—and trust me, I will—I need to know your type. In the remainder of this chapter I describe each type and subtype of hair. To make it even easier, I've included photos of each type. Examine the descriptions, then take a good look at the corresponding photo that most resembles your hair in its natural state. Don't worry if the last time you went natural was in the fifth grade. Look at the untreated roots of your hair. You'll need at least an inch of new growth to tell.

Whether you're a Type 1 or a Type 4, each strand of hair is comprised of cuticle, or fiber, layers. If you put a cross section of a hair shaft under a microscope, it would look something like the inside of a tree trunk, where you can see layer upon layer. The cuticles act as a buffer from the elements and all the damage that you inflict upon the strand. The more cuticles you have, the stronger your hair actually is.

type I : straight hair

Type 1A hair tends to be fine and thin and supersoft, with a high-octane shine.

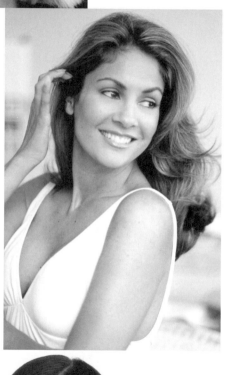

Type 1B hair is medium-textured with a lot of body.

oes your hair have absolutely no curl and no wave? You're a Type 1, which means you've got industrial-strength hair that shines and shines and shines but generally won't hold a curl. Think of Cher and actresses Helen Hunt and Joan Chen. Type 1 hair is more likely to be oily than dry, and because it has more cuticle layers than any other hair type, it's almost impossible to damage. Of course, I've seen a few Type 1s who have managed to beat the odds, usually through overprocessing with perms and bleach. Damaged Type 1 hair is very dry and brittle, with paper-thin ends. It's not a pretty sight.

Not all Type 1s are created alike. Indeed, this category contains three subtypes: A, fine and thin; B, medium-textured; and C, coarse. Type 1A hair is supersoft, with a high-octane shine. It's difficult to get this hair to do what you want. Type 1B hair has a lot of body, while Type 1C hair is the most resistant to curling and shaping.

Coarse, Type 1C hair is the most resistant to curling and shaping.

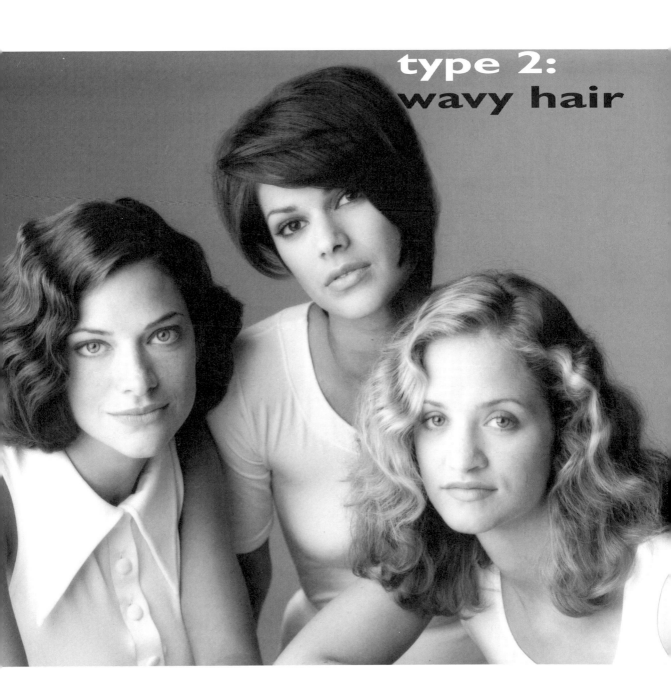

type 2:
wavy hair

Type 2A hair is fine and thin. It's easy to handle, taking on straighter or curlier styles with ease.

t ype 2 hair falls into the great divide between Type 1, straight hair, and Type 3, curly hair. A relatively unusual type, wavy hair tends to be coarse, with a definite "S" pattern to it. By that I mean the wave forms throughout the hair in the shape of the letter "S." Your hair is wavy, or Type 2, if it curves in the "S" shape while laying flat against the scalp, instead of standing away from the head the way curly hair does. Supermodel Yasmeen Ghauri, actress/model Isabella Rossellini and actress Jennifer Aniston of *Friends* (the one who sparked a craze for the ubiquitous "*Friends* haircut" of the mid-1990s) are all Type 2s. Type 2s are often confused with Type 3s because it is easy to get curly hair to lay flat and look wavy. But don't be fooled: you can't get Type 2 hair to look like Type 3 without a lot of work. Why? The hallmark of wavy hair is that it sticks close to the head: even if you cut it in layers, it won't bounce up. Again, there are three Type 2 subtypes: A, fine and thin; B, medium-textured; and C, thick and coarse. Type 2A is very easy to handle, pliantly blowing out into a straighter style or taking on curlier looks with relative ease. Types 2B and 2C hair are a little more resistant to styling and have a tendency to frizz.

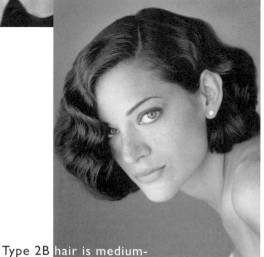

Type 2B hair is medium-textured; its waves tend to hug the head.

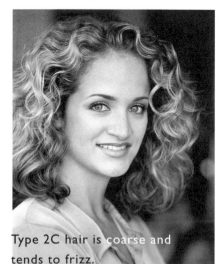

Type 2C hair is coarse and tends to frizz.

type 3: curly hair

With curly hair, there is a definite loopy "S" pattern. Pluck out a hair, stretch it out. Notice the curvy lines. Looks like a stretched-out Slinky, doesn't it? Most people think curly hair is coarse, but actually it is usually baby soft and very fine in texture—there's just a lot of it. Because the cuticle layers don't lie as flat, curly hair isn't as shiny as straight or wavy hair. The hair doesn't have a very smooth surface, so light doesn't reflect off of it as much. When curly

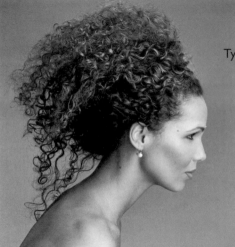

Type 3B hair grown out into long, corkscrew curls.

hair is wet, it usually straightens out. As it dries, it absorbs the water and contracts to its curliest state. Those of you with Type 3 hair know all too well that humidity makes curly hair even curlier, or even frizzier.

If you're a Type 3, your hair has a lot of body and is easily styled in its natural state, or it can be easily straightened with a blow-dryer into a smoother style. Healthy Type 3 hair is shiny, with soft, smooth curls and strong elasticity. The curls are well defined and springy: pull out a strand of hair and stretch it; it won't snap in two. Damaged Type 3 hair is usually frizzy, dull, hard and dry to the touch, with fuzzy, ill-defined curls.

Shiny, loose curls are the hallmark of Type 3A hair.

Natural, unprocessed Type 3B hair in a supershort cut.

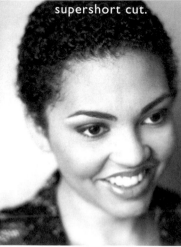

There are two subtypes of curly hair. Type 3A, hair that is very loosely curled like Julia Roberts's or Susan Sarandon's, is usually very shiny with big curls. The shorter the hair, the straighter it gets. The longer the hair, the more defined the curl. Type 3B, on the other hand, is hair with a medium amount of curl, ranging from bouncy ringlets—think of Shirley Temple and Nicole Kidman—to tight corkscrews—think of actress Cree Summer of television's *Sweet Justice* or jazz singer Cleo Laine. It's not unusual to find both subtypes coexisting on the same head. In fact, curly hair usually consists of a combination of textures, with the crown being the curliest part.

type 4: **kinky hair**

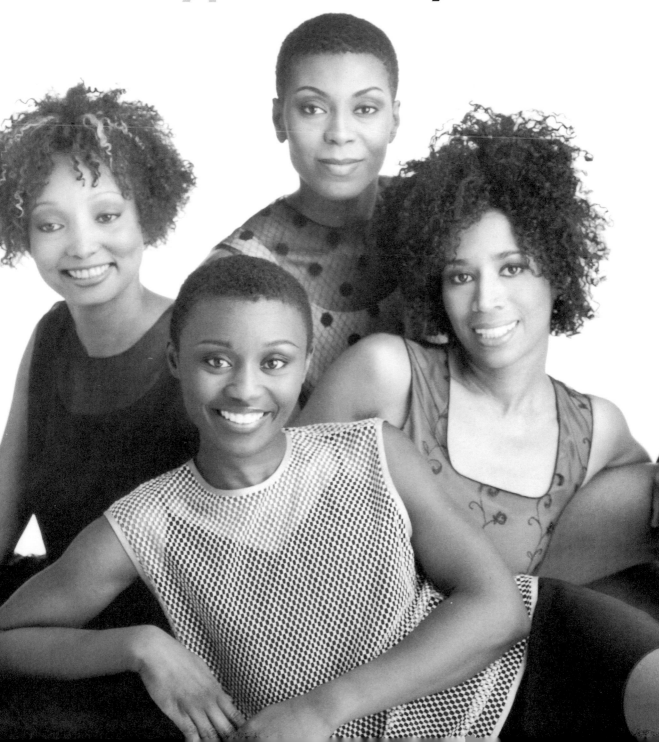

f your hair falls into the Type 4 category, then it is kinky, or very tightly curled. Generally, Type 4 hair is very wiry, very tightly coiled and very, very fragile. Like Type 3 hair, Type 4 hair appears to be coarse, but it is actually quite fine, with lots and lots of thin strands densely packed together. Healthy Type 4 hair won't shine, but it will have sheen. It will be soft to the touch and will pass the strand test with ease. It will feel more silky than it will look shiny. Oprah, Whoopi Goldberg and the actress Angela Bassett are all Type 4s.

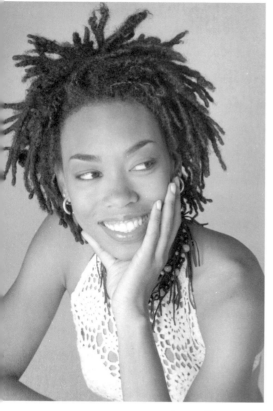

Type 4 hair looks tough and durable, but looks can be deceiving. If you have Type 4 hair, you already know that it is the most fragile hair around. Why? Type 4 hair has fewer cuticle layers than any other hair type, which means that it has less natural protection from the damage you inflict by combing, brushing, curling, blow-drying and straightening it. The more cuticle layers in a single strand of hair, the more protection it has from damage. Each time you damage your hair—fire up the curling iron, fry it with chemicals—you break down a cuticle layer, robbing your hair of much-needed moisture. I cannot emphasize this enough. It's like taking a wire and bending it again and again. Eventually, it's going to snap and break.

Many women with Type 4 hair rely on chemical relaxers to make hair easier to control. In its natural state, sometimes Type 4 hair doesn't grow very long because every time you comb it, it breaks. (Of course, if you have dreadlocks and never comb them or keep them braided, your hair can and does grow quite long.)

There are two subtypes of Type 4 hair: Type 4A, tightly coiled hair that, when stretched, has an "S" pattern, much like curly hair; and Type 4B, which has a "Z" pattern, less of a defined curl pattern (instead of curling or coiling, the hair bends in sharp angles like the letter "Z"). Type 4A tends to have more moisture than Type 4B, which will have a wiry texture. But what if your hair has been chemically straightened? How

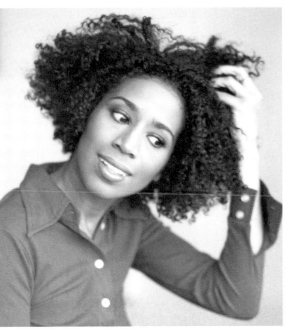

Tightly coiled Type 4A hair grown out for a full, bouncy effect.

can you tell which subtype you belong to if your hair is relaxed? You'll need at least one inch of new growth to tell. Pull at the roots. If you can see a definite curl pattern, then it's an A; if not, then it's a B.

There, that wasn't too difficult, was it? Are you still with me? Good. Because in the next chapter I'm going to tell you what to do with your uniquely beautiful type.

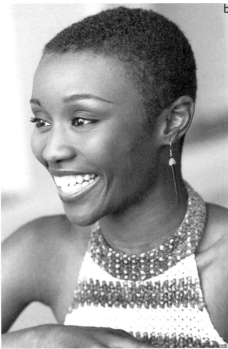

Left in its natural state, Type 4B hair has a "Z" pattern with sharp angles rather than tight curls. Here, it's shown cut into a short, natural style.

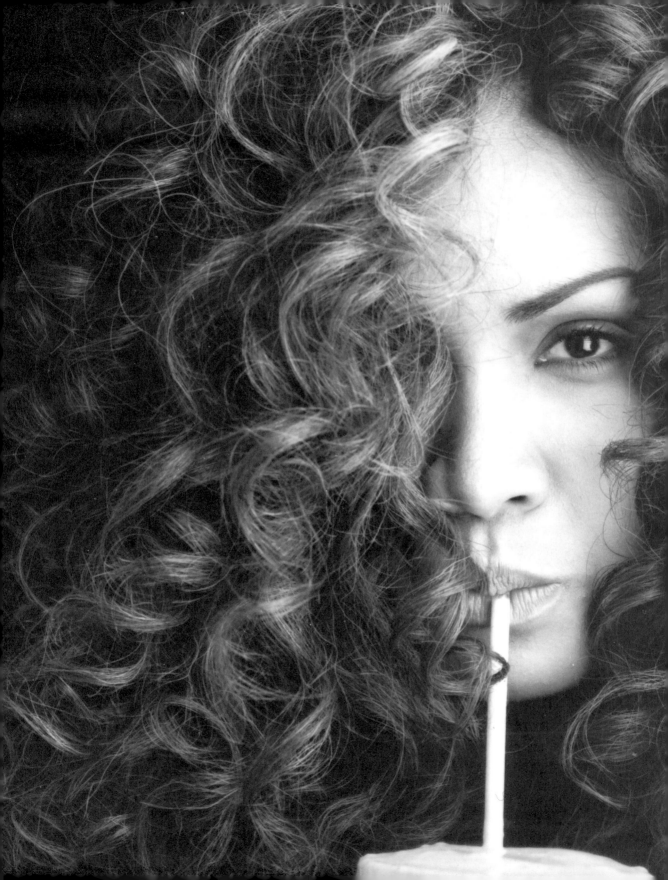

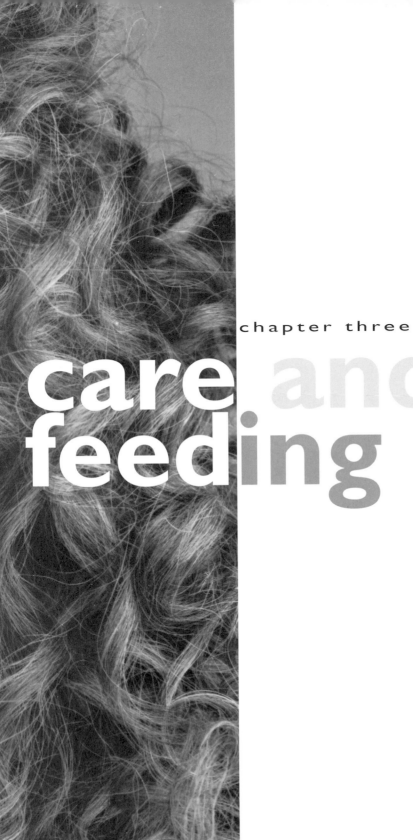

care and feeding

pampering
your hair type

More than ten years ago, before I ever took a comb to her head, I sent Oprah Winfrey flowers and a note saying, "I'm dying to get my hands in your hair." I wooed her. I'd been watching her show for some time—before it was ever syndicated, before anyone outside Chicago ever knew who she was—and I knew that she needed me. OK, maybe that sounds a little conceited, but I thought that she was an attractive woman in search of a look. She had a thick head of healthy hair; she just needed somebody to show her what to do with it. And I wanted to be that somebody.

After Oprah received my flowers, I was invited to style her hair for one show. I was a little nervous, because I wanted to do a good job. The scene at the studio didn't make me any calmer. Oprah didn't say much to me as I styled her hair. When I finished, she said she liked it—and that was it, until I got a phone call from her secretary later that day, asking me if I could come back for an encore the following morning. Of course I said yes. The following day, I styled her hair again. Again, Oprah thanked me. And again, that was it—until I got another phone call from her secretary, asking me if I could return for yet another encore. Of course I said yes. The next day, the same thing happened, and the next day, and the next day. This routine went on for over two weeks until Oprah asked me to come on board permanently.

Since then, my daily routine with her hasn't varied much. Every day, she's in my chair by 7:30 A.M. Because she works out so much, we wash her Type 4B hair— she has very coarse, thick hair with a zigzag pattern—every other day using a protein moisturizing shampoo and conditioner containing botanical ingredients. (On alternate days, I just style her hair dry with a curling iron.) Then I blow-dry her hair straight, using a hot dryer turned on high to seal the cuticle so that the hair dries shiny and smooth (otherwise her hair will frizz). Also, I don't use any of those thermal protector sprays that you see in the stores. Why? I just don't believe that there's any cosmetic out there that can protect your hair from a 1,200-watt blow-dryer and a curling iron that's so hot it can scorch your fingers. What *will* protect the hair is the proper use of blow-dryers and other heating appliances. But I'm getting ahead of myself. More on that later.

After Oprah's hair is dry, I pin it off her face and let the makeup artist go to work. While he applies the powder and paint, we shoot the breeze, gossiping about everything from the outrageous story on last night's news to whether or not she should use golden beige damask slipcovers on her new sofa to looking at runway videos of the latest fashions. Half an hour later I'm back at her hair (by now the producer is briefing her on the day's activities), this time bending a little shape into it with a hot curling iron. I curl it quickly, turning the barrel once through a strand of hair and then flipping it out again, just as quickly, making sure that I don't keep the iron in the hair for more than a few seconds. This way, the iron doesn't have a chance to cook her hair. Finally, I comb her hair through using my fingers—you don't always have to use a comb to style hair—and she's ready to go. No need for

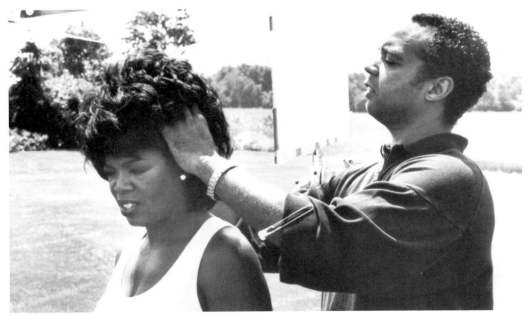

George Burns, © 1996, Harpo Productions, Inc.

hairspray unless we're going for a curlier look that requires a firmer hold. The whole process, not counting the thirty-minute session with the makeup artist, takes about forty minutes. It's easy. And Oprah always looks great—if I do say so myself.

Now, I know that you're not going to have me standing in your bathroom every morning, making sure that you look as polished as Oprah does before you head out the door. But I can let you in on my tricks of the trade so that you can look just as good. (Later on in the book, I'll help you find a hairstylist that you can trust *and* afford.)

To have great-looking hair, you don't need to spend ridiculous amounts of time on your hair. Of course, the amount of time you spend depends on whether or not you're working against your type. If you're blow-drying it straight, or setting it in electric curlers to make it curly, obviously you're going to spend more time on it than you would with a wash-and-wear 'do. I believe in picking the path of least resistance when it comes to your hair. But that's a personal decision. As long as you look good, you're not damaging your hair and your beauty routine works for you, that's all that matters.

The trick is to come up with a routine that works. As I discussed in the last chapter, a great haircut is the foundation of your look. But if your hair is dull, damaged, dirty or greasy, it won't matter how fabulous your cut is. No one will notice it—they'll be distracted by your less-than-healthy hair. Oprah's hair looks good because she's got an unbeatable combination: a flattering cut, healthy locks and an easy-does-it beauty routine. People often ask me how she keeps her mane so healthy despite subjecting it to almost daily attacks from deadly heat appliances. It's simple: conditioners, conditioners, conditioners. She's well-informed about the care and feeding of her hair; being well-informed is crucial to keeping your hair healthy and soft. And I'm going to help you get there.

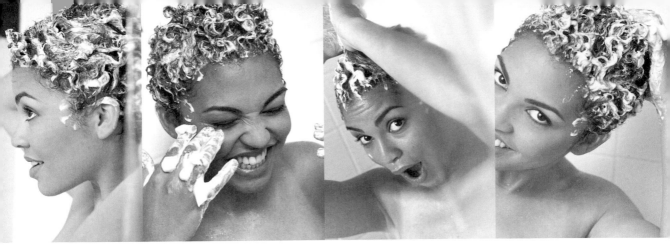

shampooing

ll hair needs to be shampooed regularly, no matter what your type. End of story. It's a myth that daily washing will dry hair out. It's a myth that daily shampoos will make hair oilier. Plain and simple, shampooing hair washes away dirt and oils and actually returns moisture to the hair. If you don't shampoo it, styling products and other debris start to build up, clogging the hair follicles and preventing vital nutrients from reaching the hair and scalp.

When that happens, it's not attractive. Let me tell you about Cindy, a regular client of mine. Once, between my crazy schedule and hers, Cindy couldn't come in to see me for several weeks. She wasn't thrilled with styling her relaxed hair on her own, so she simply didn't shampoo her hair until I could squeeze her in for an appointment. By the time she sat in my chair and I pulled a comb through her tresses, Cindy's hair was disgusting: filled with oily white flakes and emitting a *very* unpleasant odor. She was embarrassed, and I felt bad for her. After that, she never pushed things that far again; I convinced her that going so long without a shampoo couldn't be healthy for her hair. Think about it. I can wash my car in the morning, and by the end of the same day, it will have a fine layer of dust on it. If that much dirt and debris can accumulate on my *car* in one day, imagine what is happening to your hair over an extended period of time.

Of course, just how frequently you need to shampoo depends on your type. In the past, you'd flip through a beauty magazine and decide your hair type/shampoo schedule based on whether it was normal, oily or dry. It's not quite that simple. No two types are created alike, but your hair texture and how you style it will play a role in how often it needs to be shampooed. Let me explain. Type 1 hair tends to look oilier than the other types simply because the hair falls from the head in one straight line, making it easier for nutrients to slide down it and attract attention. You can be a Type 4 and have an oily scalp, but it almost always looks and feels dry because the hair's kinks and coils prevent nutrients from the scalp from distributing evenly throughout the hair. So there's never a need for anyone to oil the scalp; instead, it creates a vicious cycle. The oil clogs the hair follicles, making it even harder for the hair to get those natural lubricating oils and nutrients, which makes the hair even drier, which means you end up oiling the scalp even more. (The solution to this dilemma is more moisture, not more oil, but I'm getting ahead of myself again.)

So if you're a Type 1A with fine, limp hair, then you almost always have to shampoo daily, especially if you're going for that fluffy, bouncin' and behavin' effect. Daily sudsings with the appropriate shampoo will give your hair volume. What do I mean by appropriate? A gentle shampoo that's specified for oily hair or for daily use. Look for ingredients like tea tree oil, sage oil and chamomile. Don't use a conditioning shampoo; they deposit a slick film on the hair, weighing it down and making it even softer. With this type hair, you want the opposite effect: a shampoo that quite literally will leave your locks squeaky clean. The cleaner your hair is, the more body it will have, so forget about those shampoos that promise to give your hair body. Just use one that promises to get your hair clean. That's really all you need.

Types 1B and 1C, medium and coarse textures, have more body and should be washed either every day or every other day with a gentle shampoo. Some people think that their hair looks better when it's a "day old," a day after washing it. But if the hair tends to be oily, by all means, scrub it daily. How can you tell if it's oily?

Your hair looks greasy; it's slick to the touch and to the eye. Type 1 hair is rarely dry—unless it's very coarse or is color treated. In that case, it benefits from a good moisturizing shampoo formulated for chemically treated hair every other day.

Type 2 hair tends to be normal, neither oily nor dry. Generally, all it needs is daily to every-other-day shampoos with a product formulated for normal hair. Finding a shampoo that says "for normal hair" is a little tricky these days, what with all these "miracle" shampoos out there that claim to do everything from giving your hair "energizing body" to balancing your checkbook. Just look for a frequent-use shampoo that smells good (after all, you have to live with the scent until the next shampoo) and will clean your hair without stripping it dry. Period.

Curly Type 3 hair needs to be kept as moist as possible; when it dries out, it starts to break. Generally, if you're wearing your Type 3 hair natural, it should be washed every three days or so with a moisturizing shampoo, but it should be rinsed daily to keep the hair moist and to let the curls spring back after a night of tossing and turning in your bed. I'm a Type 3 myself, and I find that daily shampoos leave my hair a little too frizzy. My hair looks best a day or two postshampoo, when the oils have had a chance to build up a bit and calm the curls down. But on days that I skip the shampoo, I always rinse my hair in the shower; it keeps my hair fresh and removes product buildup.

If you're wearing your hair blown-dry straight, you might find that it appears to get oilier faster. In that case, step up the shampoos. Never pile hair on top of your head to shampoo. Squeeze a small amount of shampoo—about the size of a dime to a quarter, depending on your hair length—and gently stroke it through your wet hair and scalp. Rinse, rinse, rinse. You won't usually need a second scrubbing. (This applies for all hair types, by the way.)

Type 4 hair must be shampooed at least once a week. Personally, I prefer twice-weekly shampoos for this hair type, and even more often than that if you've got an

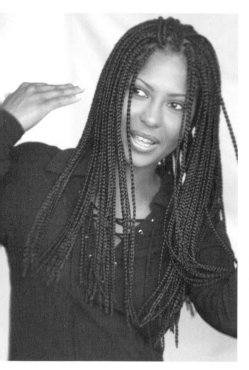

active lifestyle. As I said before, shampooing adds much-needed moisture to the hair. Why? You're wetting the hair. Water is the ultimate moisturizer. Oprah's hair always looks and feels the driest when it needs a good shampoo. Not just any shampoo will do for this type. You need a good protein-based shampoo with natural ingredients that will cleanse the hair without robbing it of moisture. Because your hair is made up of protein, adding more protein strengthens and builds elasticity into the hair shaft. So look for a protein-based shampoo that contains shea butter, glycerin, sulfur or carotene. Read the label; protein should be one of the first ingredients listed. If your hair is relaxed, look for products formulated for dry or chemically treated hair.

Natural hair that's cropped short can be shampooed daily; longer natural hair won't need to be shampooed as frequently. If you've got braids or dreadlocks, wash them as you would ordinarily, paying special attention to the scalp. Follow up by putting water-diluted conditioner in a spray bottle and spritzing the mixture on your braids. Or buy one of the many "braid sheen" sprays available on the market. Dreadlocks, in particular, need to be lubricated with oil to keep them from getting too hard and breaking off.

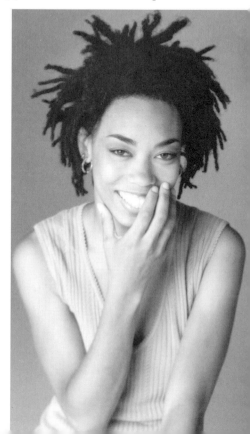

A final note: all hair, regardless of type, benefits from a good clarifying shampoo every six weeks or so. It removes buildup and returns shine and life to your hair. Follow up with a good conditioner afterward. Which brings us to . . .

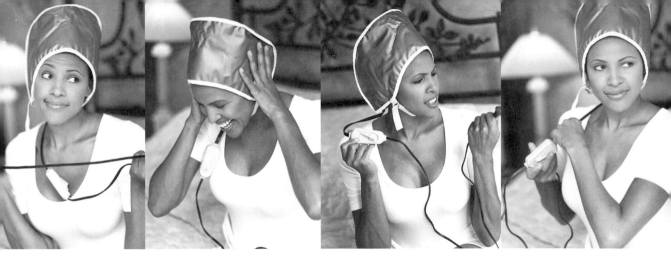

conditioning

good conditioner can forgive a lot of sins; it can strengthen damaged hair and keep healthy hair from *getting* damaged. It works by moisturizing and adding protein to the hair shaft. What it cannot do is repair hair that has already been damaged, although it can stop the abuse in its tracks. Once the hair's been damaged, however, there's nothing you can do to make it as healthy as it once was—except cut off the damage and start all over again.

Because it tends to be drier, Type 4 hair needs the most attention to conditioning treatments. Conditioners will strengthen kinky hair by keeping it moist and supple and therefore less likely to snap under pressure. Deep-condition hair twice a month; if your hair is relaxed or color-treated, make sure it is a restructuring conditioner that strengthens the hair. Following every shampoo, use a moisturizing conditioner with ingredients like lanolin and protein. Moisture is the key word here. People think hot-oil treatments moisturize the hair, but they don't. How could they? Oil and water do not mix. All a hot-oil treatment does is lubricate the hair, making it a little softer and shinier. But it will never saturate the hair with moisture.

Type 3 hair follows a similar conditioning regimen. Like Type 4 hair, you want to keep it moist. Depending on how damaged the hair may be, deep-condition it either once or twice a month. When you do, use a heat-activated penetrating conditioner; heat swells the hair shaft, making it easier for conditioners to penetrate. Use a heat cap or a hooded dryer with a plastic bag. Don't have either? Run hot water—as hot as you can stand—over a towel and wrap it around your head, leaving it on for twenty minutes. (Type 2s, 4s and damaged 1s can do this as well.) If your hair is healthy, you won't need to condition it during your in-between-shampoo rinses in order to untangle it.

Types 1 and 2 hair require much lighter conditioning. Type 1 hair needs a moisturizing conditioner only once a month to keep it in shape, while Type 2 hair benefits from a once-a-week moisturizing session. Tame dry, bushy Type 2 and flyaway Type 1 locks with a "finishing" rinse, which is just a fancy name for the good old-fashioned cream rinse/detangler.

don't believe the hype

Over the years, Terry has finally found the perfect styling products to control her Type 3 hair—a mixture of leave-in conditioner and lightweight gel. The combination works for her, leaving her curls shiny and frizz-free. But is she satisfied with the status quo? Of course not. Terry's a product victim, haunting drugstores and beauty supply stores, endlessly searching for the perfect product—anything that claims to be a straightening balm, defrizzer, no-frizzer, curl enhancer, curl flattener . . . you get the picture. She believes the hype. The products never work, so they're currently taking up space in her bathroom for all her guests to experiment with. Meanwhile, she returns again and again to her tried-and-true formula, broker but not wiser.

Still, finding the perfect styling product is a trial-by-error proposition. There are hundreds upon hundreds of products out there; only a handful—or maybe just one—will work for your hair. Something might work for someone who appears to have the same exact type hair as you but fail miserably on your own tresses. A curl

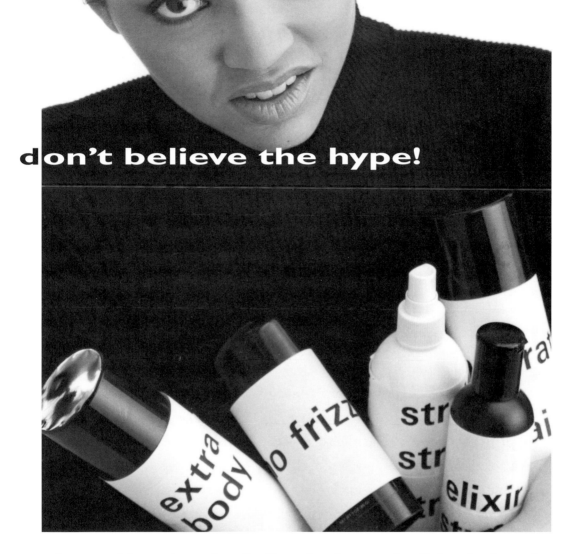

don't believe the hype!

enhancer might work wonders for Terry, but for you, that little miracle worker actually might be a moisturizing hand and body lotion. That's right, *lotion*. There's nothing wrong with dabbing a little on your hair. If it moisturizes your locks and gives you the look you want, then go for it. Many of the ingredients are identical to that expensive hair cream that's currently busting your budget. Look for a body lotion that contains natural ingredients like aloe vera, wheat protein, glycerin, and vitamin E. (Type 1s with ultrafine hair should skip this trick.)

Don't get me wrong; I believe every type benefits from the finishing polish that styling products can give the hair. Even if you've got the ultimate in minimalism— a crew cut—a little dab of pomade or gel polishes off your cut, adding interest and texture to even the most ordinary 'dos. The trick is knowing which goop is going to best work for your hair.

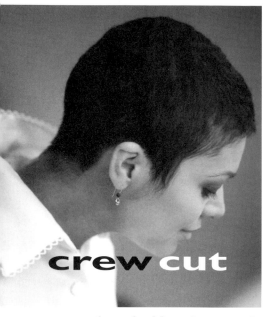

crew cut

This isn't always the easiest proposition. Enter any beauty supply store and there are literally dozens upon dozens of different gels, mousses, defining lotions, shine enhancers and other products crammed onto the shelves. There are products out there that promise to fight frizz, straighten hair without chemicals, undamage the damaged, thicken the thin, seal the split, add shine, enhance color, put in curl, take out curl, sculpt it, protect it from the sun, protect it from the blow-dryer . . . the list goes on and on. Apparently, the folks making this stuff never heard about truth in advertising.

We've all seen the ads for the product that promises to "ease" frizz. (No names!) They all feature dramatic before-and-after photos. In the before shot, the models sport whacked-out, Bride of Frankenstein hair and sad-sack faces. In the after shot, the frizz has been transformed into glossy ringlets and the models look like they just won the lottery—all thanks to the magic product. (Oh, please!) I know women who ran—*ran*—to the store because they couldn't wait to try this product. And it didn't work. Why? Because my friends didn't have that little something that the models in the photos *did* have: a hairdresser styling and setting their curls just so, right before the photographer clicked the camera. These antifrizz products contain dimethicone, a silicone-based substance that can add shine but does little else to the hair. (Except make it look really greasy if you use too much.)

And then there was that infamous hair relaxer sold through infomercials that promised to give women straight hair "naturally"—without chemicals. This product was supposed to be so good for your hair that you could apply it over your old relaxer. The result? Dozens upon dozens of women literally lost their hair—some of them permanently. The company went out of business in the wake of lawsuits. But all the money in the world can't replace your precious hair.

My point is, if the product sounds too good to be true, you can bet you're going to waste your hard-earned money if you buy it. Most of the products out there are dreamed up by clever marketing professionals dead set on getting you to buy, buy, buy. The fact is, gels, mousses, pomades and setting lotions can alter the look of your hair slightly, maybe even make it a little easier to control, but they're not going to make dramatic changes in your hair texture.

So beware before you buy a shampoo that purports to thicken your hair. It can't, so it won't. But as I said, you *can* use gels and mousses that coat the hair a little and give it a little extra oomph. Mousse doesn't provide as much hold as gel, but it works well for baby-soft Type 1 hair in need of a lift. For natural, not stiff-looking, volume, squirt mousse (about the size of a golf ball) into your hands, distribute it through the roots of your hair and then blow-dry. (Applying products *after* blow-drying will just flatten the hair.)

While those "relaxing balms" that claim to straighten hair might make it a little easier to blow-dry, that's about all they can do. Using them repeatedly can actually cause buildup that can damage your hair. But if you want to control frizz, some heavier gels can and do weigh the hair down, making it look a little less voluminous.

In general, it's a good idea to avoid styling products that contain alcohol. Alcohol will dry hair out, so that over time you'll be left with a head full of straw. There is one case in which alcohol actually makes a product perform better: holding hairsprays. Hairsprays, which contain "memory" resins that hold your style in place, require alcohol. Why? Non-alcohol-based holding sprays spritz on wet, making your hair revert to its natural texture. Curly hair will frizz; straight or relaxed locks will flop. Alcohol-based hairsprays dry quickly on the hair, preserving the style and desired texture of the hair. Still, I'm not fond of them, and I rarely use them on Oprah's hair. If you must use them, prevent product buildup by using a good clarifying shampoo afterward. Never comb or brush hair after styling products have dried on it; you'll risk breaking your hair. Wet hair first before combing. And re- member: with a good haircut as your base, you won't need a lot of styling products to maintain your hairstyle.

homemade help

Some of you will be tempted to pinch pennies by whipping up a conditioning concoction at home. Proceed cautiously: store-bought products have been tested for effectiveness in a laboratory; homemade concoctions have not. I believe that store-bought products are superior, but in a pinch, there are a few things you can try. For dry, brittle hair, give yourself a hot-oil treatment with olive oil. Pour about half a cup in a small glass, then put the glass in a saucepan filled with water. Heat the oil until it is warm, but not scalding, to the touch. Apply the oil to your hair, wrap your hair in a warm towel and leave it set for twenty minutes to half an hour. Then shampoo. The oil (you can use other oils such as coconut or peanut) will add shine to the hair, lubricating it so that it is softer. But remember, an oil cannot moisturize your hair. It's also difficult to wash out, so you might end up overshampooing to compensate. The result? Hair that's even drier than when you started. This method works for some hair types; others will find it a waste of time. Inexpensive hot-oil treatment packets are more effective, since they contain oils that are lighter than anything you could find at home. Because the oils are lighter, they are easier to wash out.

Mayonnaise is fine to try as well; the cholesterol from the vegetable oils and egg yolks conditions the hair and adds protein. Again, mayonnaise won't do anything to moisturize your hair, since it is mainly an oil. Apply it to your hair and let it set for about half an hour, then shampoo. Another trick to try is mashed-up avocado. (Make sure to skin the avocado first!) Avocado contains vitamins A, C, D and E and potassium, ingredients that are good for your hair. It will soften, lubricate and add a nice touch and feel to your hair. Mash a very ripe avocado in a bowl and apply the pulp to your hair. Wrap your hair in a plastic bag and leave the avocado in overnight to penetrate the hair. Follow with a light moisturizing shampoo—and make sure you get all the avocado out. Be careful about using a heat cap on these homemade conditioners; you don't want to end up with hair that smells like cooked food.

one more thing

prefer products that contain all-natural botanical ingredients. I'm no chemist, but in my experience, botanical ingredients leave the hair looking and feeling better. Products containing all-natural ingredients are more expensive to process than products containing synthetic ingredients, so obviously they are going to cost more. Three-dollar shampoos are not going to be "all natural"—how could they be so cheap without some cost-cutting synthetic ingredients tossed in there? I'm not saying that synthetic products are bad for your hair; I just think that they're not as good as those containing botanical ingredients like chamomile, comfrey and rosemary.

Of course, these days, just about everyone is on a budget, so I know that sometimes it's hard to justify spending twenty dollars on a conditioner. You don't have to go broke caring for your hair; still, I believe that you do get what you pay for. So watch the bottom line, but do spend as much as you can afford on quality hair-care products. Just be smart about it. Do a little sleuthing, and look at enthusiastic advertising claims with a skeptical eye; ask your stylist for help in your search. Trust me, very few miracle discoveries are being marketed right now. The moral of this story? Experiment by all means, but if you find something that works for you, *stick with it.*

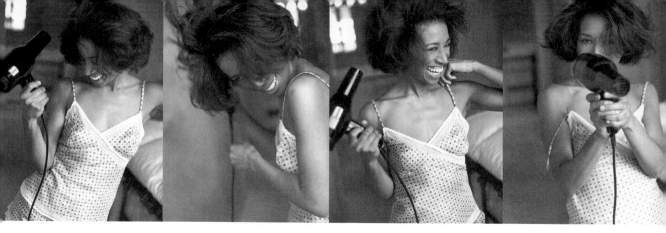

blow-drying

straightening

it's possible to blow out any texture of hair for a straight look. The tighter the curl in your hair, however, the trickier it is to do it yourself while your hair is in its natural state. Still, it's not impossible.

First of all, your hair must be clean and sopping wet; if you want to wear your hair straight, only blow-dry your hair after you've shampooed it. Blow-drying dirty hair just bakes in the dirt—a surefire recipe for damaged locks. Use a moisturizing conditioner every time you shampoo to restore elasticity to your hair. Blow-dry your hair no more than three times a week; twice a week is optimal. To start, you'll need several hairclips, a gun-type blow-dryer and either a round bristle brush or a Denman brush with plastic bristles. The larger the circumference of the round brush, the straighter your hair will be. Obviously, if your hair is supershort, it won't fit around a large brush, so pick your brush size accordingly. Flat paddle brushes are good for straight hair or wavy hair, but they won't work as well straightening Type 3 or Type 4 hair. If you're all thumbs and can't coordinate using a blow-dryer and a brush, you can get virtually the same results with a blow-dryer equipped with a brush attachment.

If your hair is medium length or longer, divide it into four sections—two on top, two on the bottom—and secure each section with a clip. Unclip one bottom section; from that section, section off a chunk of hair—say, about an inch wide. Start at the scalp, rolling the brush through the hair as the dryer follows the brush down the length of the hair to the ends, pulling the hair straight until the section is completely dry. (Make sure the dryer is at least one to two inches away from the brush.) "Dry" is the key word here. When the hair is completely dry, it will have a shine to it; if it doesn't shine, that means the hair is still damp and will dry puffy and frizzy. This is why it is important to dry one section at a time, until each section is completely dry, smooth and shiny. The heat from the blow-dryer will mold the hair like wax into whatever shape you put it. When you've completed your entire head—the process should take no more than thirty minutes for shoulder-length hair of average thickness—shake your hair out, brush it or run your fingers through it. That's all you'll need to maintain your style. If your hair is relaxed, however, it might need to be touched up with a curling iron to polish the look—unless you're deliberately going for a look that's stick straight.

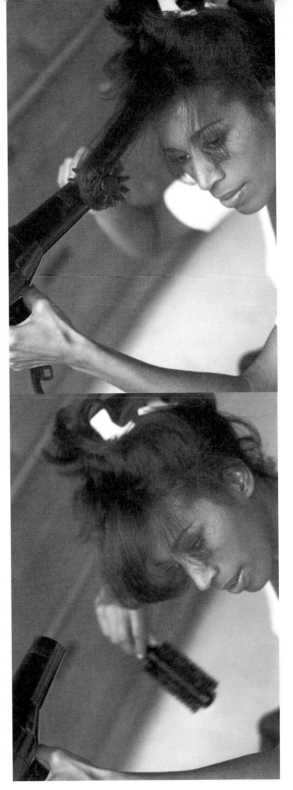

keeping the curl

If you're a curly Type 3 and want to relax some of the curl without straightening it, here's a drying trick for you. Shampoo and condition your hair and blot it with a towel until it is damp but not sopping wet, being careful not to disturb the curls. Apply your favorite styling product—gel, mousse or pomade. Let your hair air-dry until it is almost but not completely dry. Then take your blow-dryer (you can use a diffuser attachment, but it is not essential) and grab a chunk of hair. Blow the roots dry and then very, very gently pull the curls down as the dryer travels down the shafts of the hair. Be careful not to pull too hard on your hair, as doing so will straighten it too much. Continue until your entire head is completely dry. Do not section the hair off. When you're done, your curls will look longer and smoother and will have lots and lots of body.

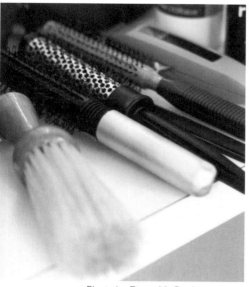

Photo by Darcy McGrath

Whichever technique you opt for, be careful out there: blow-drying your hair straight puts a lot of stress on it. You're pulling the hair when it's at its weakest—when it's wet. Don't be aggressive; blow-drying can really damage your hair. Please, please, please proceed with caution. Your hair is the only hair you've got.

blow-drying straight hair

If you want to enhance the smooth shine of your Type 1 hair, pick either a Denman brush with plastic bristles or a boar-bristle round brush. The boar-bristle brush is a good choice if you want to disguise frayed ends; it helps smooth out the hair, giving it a consistent texture while shaping the ends into the desired style.

The smaller the diameter of the brush, the more volume you'll achieve with your hair. Longer hair can achieve that swinging sixties look with a flat paddle brush.

To reduce blow-drying time, towel-dry freshly shampooed hair. If you have a simple, long, layered cut, you won't need a brush at all. Simply work the blow-dryer through your hair until your hair is dry. If you want to accentuate the smooth texture, separate your hair into four sections: two on top, two on the bottom. Start brushing each section from the roots first, working the brush down the length of the hair until it is completely dry. Aim the dryer at the moving brush, keeping it moving in the same direction as the brush. The idea is to smooth the hair out so that light will reflect it for a high-octane shine.

Spend time getting moisture out of the roots of your hair while spending as little time as possible drying the ends. A lot of people make the mistake when drying their hair of putting too much heat on the ends, which are the oldest parts of your hair. That's how damage begins; the ends don't have the same moisture content as the roots, which are the youngest part of your hair.

If your hair is shorter and layered, take big sections of it, drying a section at a time. Experiment, using different brush sizes on your hair to lock in volume and shape. Again, be gentle with your hair; don't rip the brush through it, and be careful not to get hair tangled in the brush. The less you yank on your hair, the healthier you keep it.

curling it

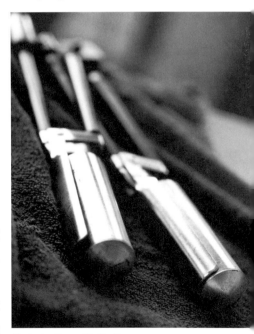

rollers are great for putting in curls—and for taking them out. If you've got Type 1 or Type 2 hair and want to add some volume, Velcro rollers are a great option. After blow-drying your hair to the point where it is almost but not completely dry, roll it with the Velcro rollers. Spritz

Photo by Darcy McGrath

with hairspray and then set the curls with a blast of heat from the blow-dryer. Remove rollers and style. This trick is great for giving fine or medium Type 1 hair some volume without a lot of bend. Since straight hair tends to be stubborn, it won't curl much, but the rollers will add some movement. If your hair is coarse, it will be even straighter and more resistant. There's also more hair to handle, so you'll need to section off smaller amounts in order to fit it on the rollers—which means that you'll have more rollers on your head. If you've got wavy hair, you can use Velcro rollers to make your hair even wavier.

I'm not fond of electric rollers at all. I think they're highly damaging and give hair a dated, overly done look. Hot rollers will not straighten curly hair. If you insist on using them, keep them in for only a minute, and be sure to use some sort of holding spray or hairspray to give more support to your curls.

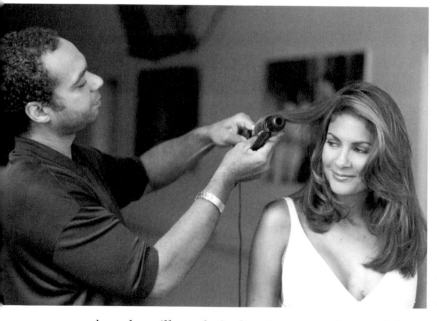

Although less damaging than hot rollers, curling irons still have the potential to hurt your hair. They're versatile, work on any hair texture and are great for adding a lot or a little curl. If you want to add just a little bend at the ends of your hair, use a big-barreled iron. The tighter the curl you're going after, the smaller the size of the barrel you'll need. Curling irons are also good for smoothing out or straightening highly textured hair, sealing the hair shaft with heat. So if your hair is very curly or kinky, you'll need a hotter curling iron formulated for textured hair.

Whatever your hair texture, it is important that you keep the curling iron in your hair for only a few seconds. Yes, *seconds*. Some people will twirl their hair around the iron and let it sit there. That cooks the hair, leaving it fried with those burned-off white ends. Section off the hair, spritzing it with a holding spray. Run the iron down the shafts of hair, twisting the ends under. Then take the iron out. This way, you're only putting heat on the hair for a matter of seconds. Continue through your entire head of hair until you have the desired effect.

Don't want to use heat on your hair but still want a curly look? Many women turn to sponge rollers. They're easy to sleep in and set the hair well, but they're horrible for your hair. The hair gets caught in the spongy texture and breaks off. If you must use them, remove the little plastic clamp—it just leaves a telltale crimp in the hair—and wrap the rollers with end paper or tissue. Roll the hair and stick a bobby pin through the hole of the sponge. You'll get a smoother set and healthier hair.

Pin curls are another option. They're easier on your hair, too.

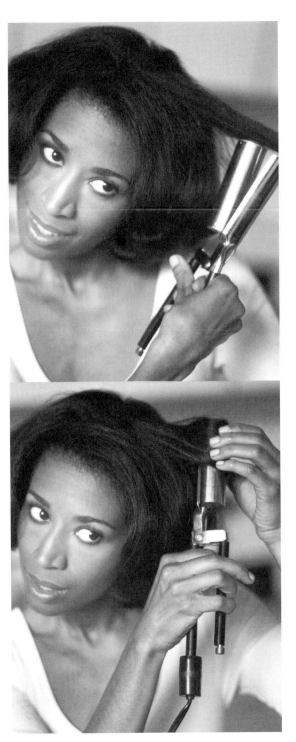

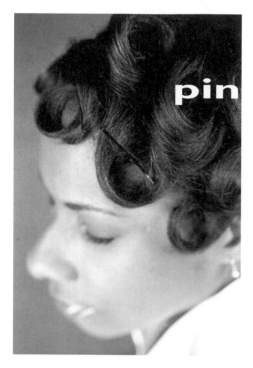

pin curls

Using end paper on the ends of the hair, wind the hair round and round itself, until it is rolled up to the scalp. Stick a bobby pin in it to secure the curl. The size of the pin curl will determine the degree of curl. It will take an hour and a half to two hours for pin curls to set on dry hair. They're easy to sleep in, and they don't damage the hair.

the wet set

Setting hair wet with old-fashioned rollers isn't antiquated. In fact, if you have textured Type 3 or Type 4 hair that you want to straighten, it's one of the easiest and most lasting ways to get hair straight—if you have the patience to do it. You use minimal heat from a dryer and you're not yanking the hair straight with a brush while using high heat. And you won't have to use a curling iron or blow-dryer once you're done. The idea is to reshape the natural curl to the size of the roller. It works well on natural Type 3 hair, loosely kinked natural Type 4 hair and relaxed Type 4 hair.

Shampoo hair and condition as usual. Apply a styling lotion while the hair is still sopping wet. The styling lotion will give the hair more control; if you want a fuller look, don't use lotion at all. If you want a straight look, use as large a roller as possible; for shoulder-length hair, use rollers the size of beer cans (or use that old standby from the sixties, frozen orange juice cans). Smaller, rod-sized rollers will just frizz the hair. Magnetic plastic rollers are the best.

Section off hair, making neat parts. Roll the top part of the head so that the rollers face backward. If the roller is two inches wide, section off a piece of hair that's the same size. Comb the hair until it is smooth, and then smooth it around the roller, starting at the ends and then rolling the hair up the scalp. Then take a roller clamp and secure the curl in place. Remember that the larger the roller, the larger the size of the curl, and vice versa. Use pronged clips to secure the rollers in place. Don't roll the hair so tight that it pulls the scalp, but don't roll it too loose either. If it's too loose, the hair will crinkle, enabling it to revert to its curly state. Dry hair under a hooded dryer until it is completely dry—a process that usually takes anywhere from an hour and a half to two or three hours. Always make sure that your hair is completely dry before removing the rollers. If it's not, you're defeating the purpose. The hair will frizz. As long as your hair dries completely around the roller, you will get a smoother, straighter look.

Another old-fashioned option is the wrap set. This works well on most types of natural Type 3 hair and on relaxed Type 4 hair only. Begin with sopping-wet hair and apply a styling lotion. With the wrap set, you will need only two large-sized rollers. Section off a chunk of hair at the crown and roll it with the two rollers, stacking one under the other. Secure them with pronged clips. Make sure the hair is rolled taut. Then take the rest of the wet hair and brush it around your head, smoothing it as you go. Secure with clips. The idea is to use your head as one giant roller, thereby straightening the hair. Sit under a dryer for about forty-five minutes until your hair is completely dry. If your hair is very thick or long, you'll need to take it down and then reroll it in the opposite direction so that the hair underneath can now dry on top. Secure with clips. Sit under the dryer until the bottom hair that's now on top is completely dry. Take your hair down, brush and you've got swingingly straight hair. (With short hair you won't need to use the rollers. Just brush it straight around your head and secure with clips.) This method is amazingly gentle on your hair, and it works.

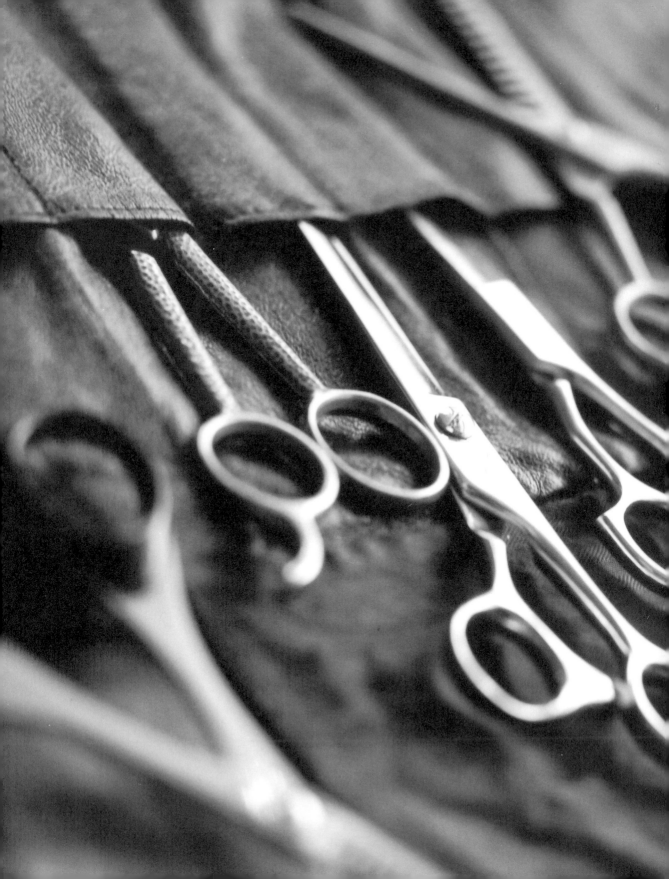

chapter four
surgery

the art of the cut

It's a miracle. A great haircut, that is. It can shave years off your age, make split ends disappear, repair damage, make too-thick hair look thinner, make too-thin hair look thicker, tame frizz, pump up the volume, make the dull shiny, and add sophistication, movement, style and pizzazz to your look. A major new haircut puts the world on notice that you've got a new attitude. Think of all the women out there who made truth out of the cliche, hacking off their locks as soon as they dumped their boyfriends—literally cutting that man right out of their hair. And many a supermodel's career has been made—or broken—by answering that age-old question plaguing many a woman: to cut or not to cut?

Think I'm overstating my point? When she first came to my salon, back in the early 1990s, Halle Berry was a young actress/model struggling to make it in Chicago. She had long, thick, layered Type 3 hair that was driving her nuts—and no wonder. The combination of hair color, relaxers and frequent blow-drying had left her hair dry and brittle. To top it off, she had a patch of hair at the crown of her head that kept breaking off, because it was twice as curly, twice as unruly and twice as fragile as the rest of her hair. (Remember, it's common for Type 3s to have several textures coexisting on one head.) To compound matters, it took her about an hour to blow-dry her hair straight every other day. She had a lot of hair to take care of, and she was ready for a change.

So I suggested that we go short—very short. She was leaving for California to audition for the pilot for a new show called *Paper Dolls.* I thought a supershort cut was just the ticket, a new image for a new life. Of course, making such a change isn't something that anyone should take lightly; we're all pretty much identified by our hair. But Halle was more than ready and told me, "Go for it." In one sitting, we cut it off. I took scissors in hand and sculpted her mane down to a neat little pixie cut. The sides and bottom were left naturally curly; the top I left a little longer. It was a versatile cut. She could blow-dry the top for a fluffy, sassy look, or she could wrap it for a sleek, Josephine Baker style, or she could do the wash-and-wear thing and let her curls go free. The cut brought out her pretty, petite features and totally eliminated any need for chemicals and lengthy blow-drying sessions. It gave her a fresh, modern look that worked with her natural hair texture, and it became her trademark. In fact, as Halle's career took off in films like *The Last Cowboy*, *The Flintstones*, *Jungle Fever* and *Losing Isaiah*, women around the country started clamoring for "the Halle Berry cut."

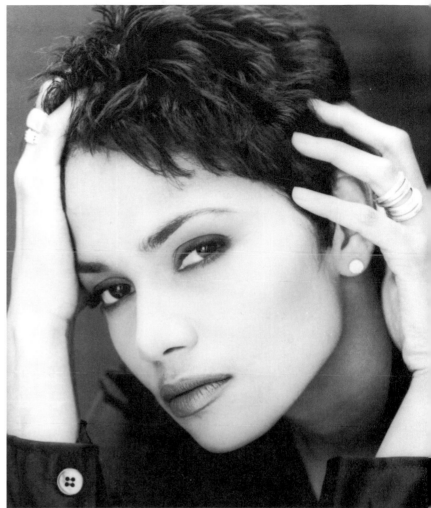

Firooz Zahedi / Botaish Group

Obviously, Halle is a beautiful, sexy, intelligent woman with plenty of talent and charisma to spare. It was her talent, and not her haircut, that made her a success. But the haircut gave her an edge. At the time, all the other young actresses were sporting long, layered hair—what I call the "anchorwoman" look. With her short haircut, Halle didn't look like anyone else out there; she was a standout. Her haircut gave her instant recognition. Today, in addition to her acting career, she's a successful model/spokeswoman, with a lucrative cosmetics contract with Revlon. You can see her looking fabulous in all those magazine ads—and she's still got that Halle Berry cut.

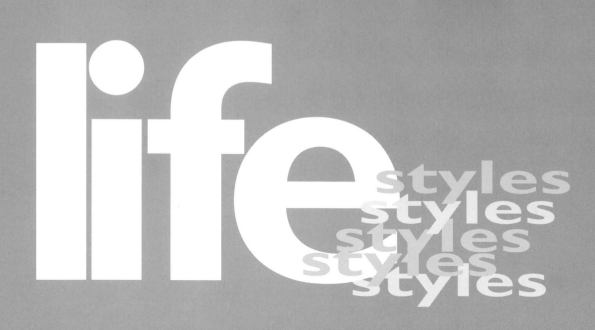

life styles styles styles styles styles

There was a time when women were slaves to their hair—and slaves to the styles of the day. Today, women have discarded old rules about how and what a "real" woman should be and do, and their attitudes toward beauty have eased up as well. To paraphrase an old song, free your mind and your hair will follow. Today, looking good is about accepting the beauty God handed out at birth. Not that you have to take the back-to-nature approach to beauty—a little gilding of the lily is good for the soul.

But enhancing what you've got doesn't mean that you have to spend a lifetime chained to a hairstylist's chair. Women today lead extraordinarily busy lives. Who has time to spend worshipping at the beauty altar? Your hair has got to get with your program and not the other way around. Which means that it should take you from the gym to the boardroom to the ballroom to a vacation for two in Aruba with ease, looking fabulous the whole time. And it can. Don't believe me? Check out the next few pages, where I've featured five women whose looks and lives I admire.

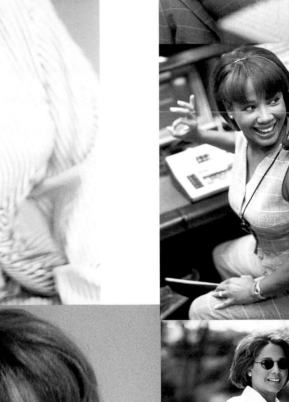

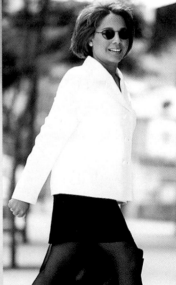

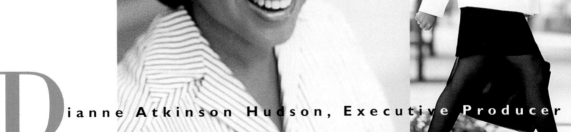

Dianne Atkinson Hudson, Executive Producer

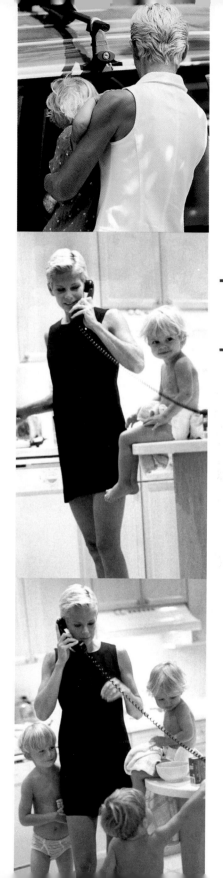

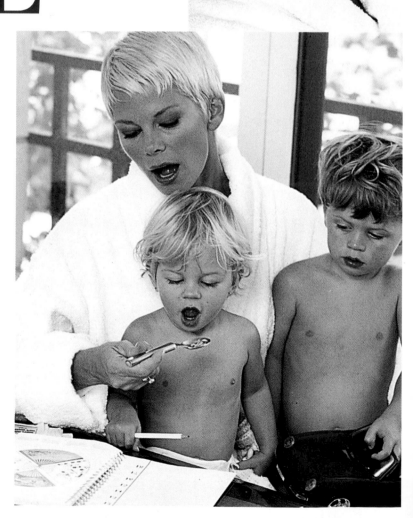

L ynn Eggers, mom

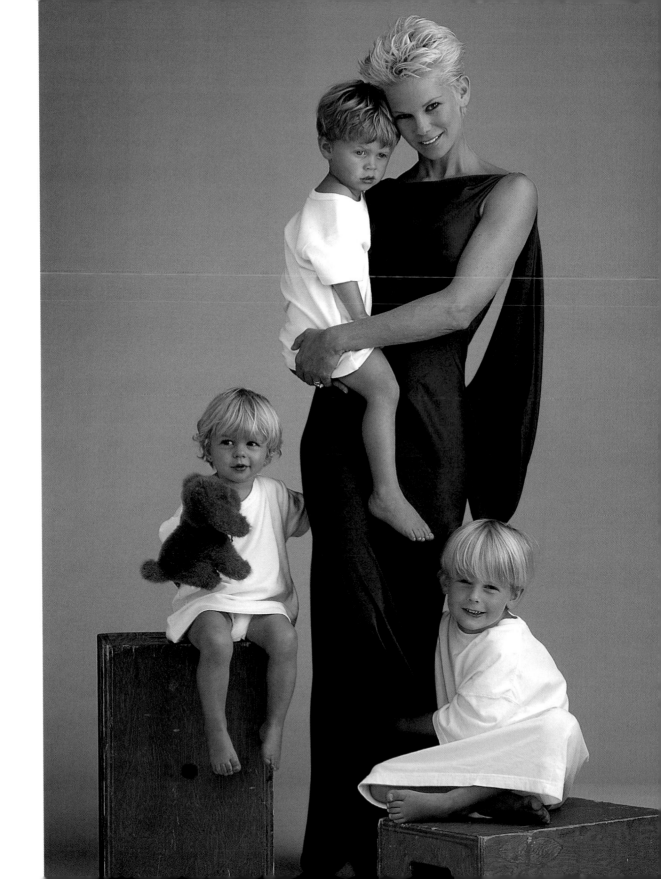

J urgita Grubeviciute, professional athlete, personal trainer

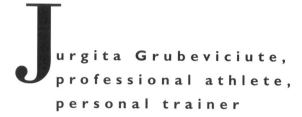

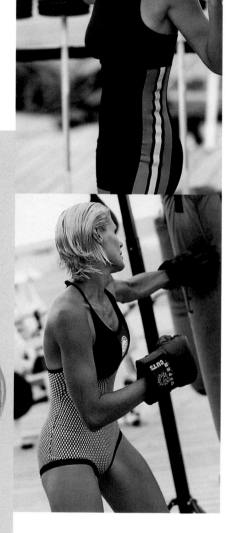

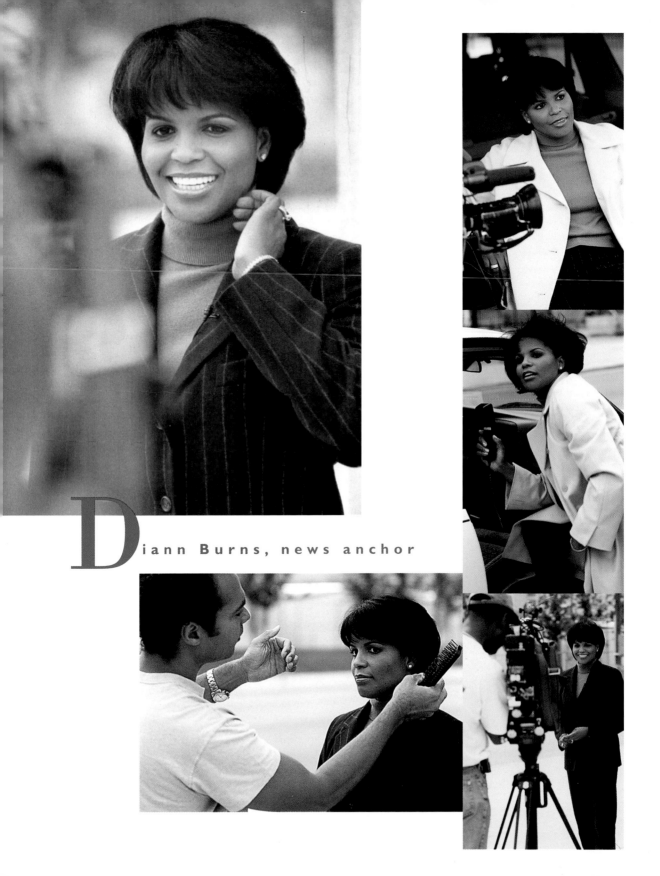

Diann **Burns,** news anchor

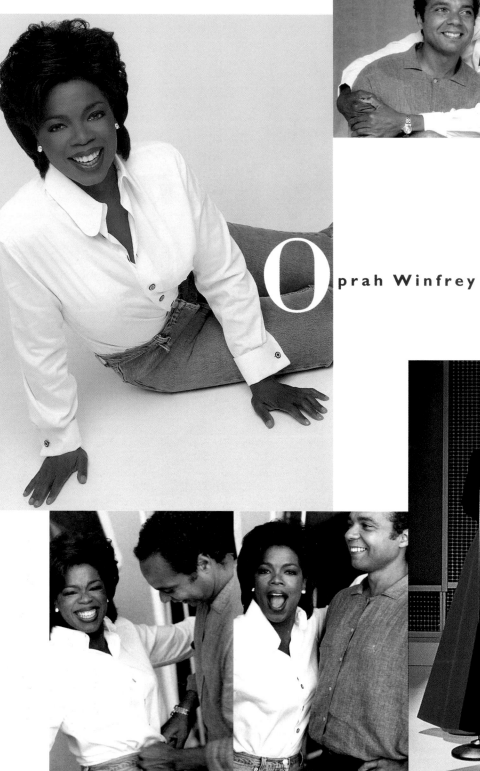

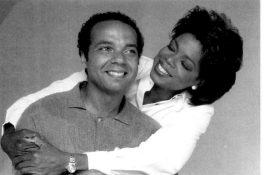

Oprah Winfrey

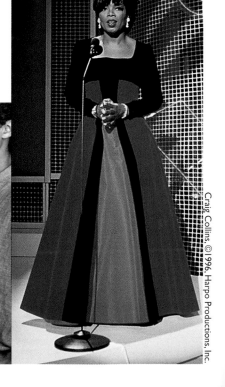

Craig Collins, © 1996, Harpo Productions, Inc.

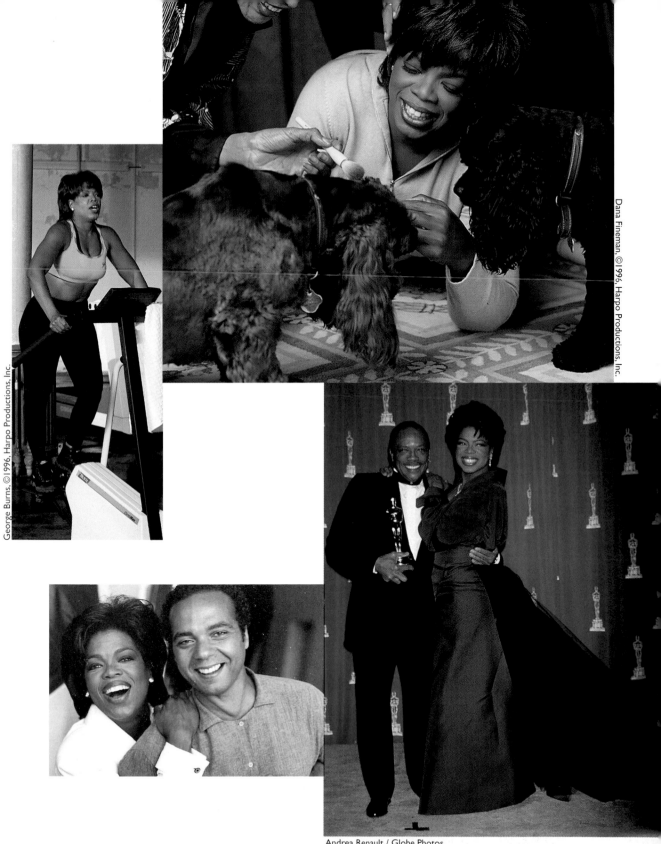

George Burns, ©1996, Harpo Productions, Inc.

Dana Fineman, ©1996, Harpo Productions, Inc.

Andrea Renault / Globe Photos

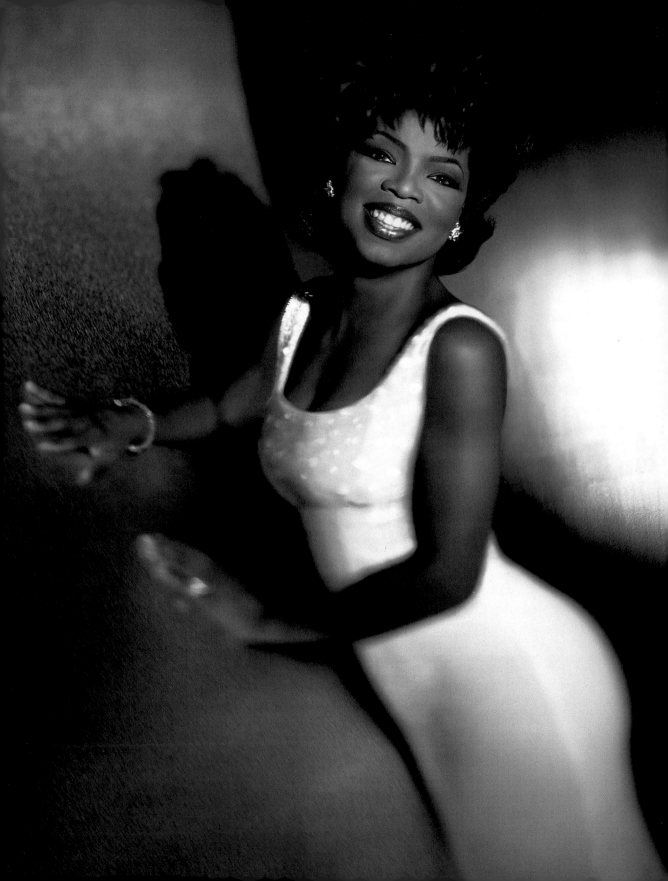

Of course, you don't have to take such a dramatic plunge, going from long to barely there, to have a flattering new look. Sometimes all it takes is a little snip here and there, or cutting bangs, or angling one side of your hair, to take your look from plain to knockout. But whether you decide to go long or short or somewhere in between, do remember that change is a good thing. One of my pet peeves is when women get stuck in the same look for decades, because they're either afraid of change or believe that they look their most beautiful in one particular style. It's a mistake to get stuck doing instant replays of a haircut you've been wearing since your senior prom. Again and again, I run into a woman who believes she was at her peak in a particular decade, and she's been wearing the same 'do ever since. It's a sad mistake, because it makes the woman look like she's not very happy with her life the way it is right now—or else why would she be stuck back in '76? It's also incredibly aging. There's a fine line between sticking with a look that works for you and getting stuck in a time warp. Some women thrive on changing their hair faster than they change their mood; others don't like to stray too much from the tried and true. But even actresses known for a signature hairstyle—for instance, Farrah Fawcett or Goldie Hawn—make little changes along the way to keep it updated.

The key is to take what you've got and work with it. I find that one of the most difficult tasks in my line of work is getting people to appreciate what they have. A good cut should simplify your life, making styling your hair a very simple proposition. I believe that a good haircut is the foundation of any look; no amount of curling, spraying, and fussing can disguise a bad haircut.

A good cut should work with your hair texture, easily falling into place with clean, clear lines, whether your hair is sleek Type 1, a curvy Type 2, a corkscrewed Type 3, or an abundantly springy Type 4. I also believe that money talks. You don't have to spend hundreds of dollars on a cut, but you can't expect to get a good cut for eight dollars at one of those cookie-cutter chains. They're trained to cut hair quickly, not well. If someone's standing over you with a pair of scissors in his hands, you want him to be looking at you, not at the clock. (Chapter 9 is all about finding the perfect stylist for you.) Another reason to avoid the cookie-cutter chains: they churn out cookie-cutter looks. Why would you want to look just like the woman sitting in the chair who had the appointment before you? The days are long gone when, for a woman to look "with it," she had to have the "it cut" of the moment (even if actress Jennifer Aniston did start a shag craze with her see-it-everywhere *Friends* cut of the mid-1990s).

Which brings me to another of my pet peeves. When it comes to hair, people aren't individual enough. They go to a salon and come out looking ridiculous, trying to keep up with the latest 'do. You see women coming out of those assembly-line beauty parlors with patent-leather hair piled three feet high. You know what I'm talking about—hair that looks like it's been sculpted and then shellacked or frozen into a mold. (I really wonder how water penetrates it.) Then there are the women who have permed their beautiful straight hair so often that it looks fried. Or those women with freeze-dried, bilevel, mall hair that's bleached and cut short on the top and hangs in a long frizzy perm on the bottom. And then there's my personal favorite: big hair that's dyed a horrible orange color and has "Howdy Do" bangs that say hello before the rest of you makes it through the door. All these "don't" 'dos are candidates for membership in what I call "Andre's Hair Hall of Shame." I'm joking, but it really is sad, because women who have hair like that get judged right away— before they ever open their mouths. No one takes them seriously.

So when you look for a new 'do, I'd like you to throw out the rule books. Forget about wearing hair in your face to make your round face look oval, forget about disguising your square jaw, forget about cutting your hair above your shoulders once you've hit forty (look at Susan Sarandon, Lauren Hutton, Diana Ross, Farrah, Goldie and Raquel Welch). Regardless of what those old beauty magazines might tell you, there is no one ideal face shape or hair type. I don't believe in blindly subscribing to hairdos with names like "The Gypsy" or "The Dorothy Hamill" or "The *Friends* Cut." Individuality is the theme song here. To make your haircut sizzle, you've got to take into account your hair texture, facial features, lifestyle and the

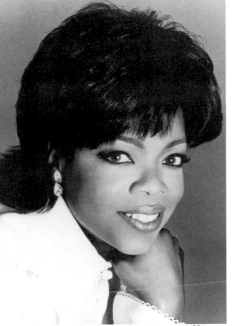

Francesco Scavullo, © 1994, Harpo Productions, Inc.

Steve Green, © 1996, Harpo Productions, Inc.

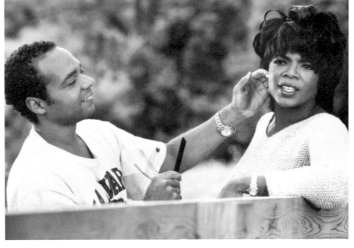

amount of time you're willing to spend on your hair.

Over the years, I've taken Oprah through dozens of hair changes. At this writing, her hair is cut in a mod shag, filled with different degrees of layers, which gives the impression of having both blunt-cut and layered hair. Because Oprah has very thick, coarse hair, I decided to remove a lot of the weight and bulk by cutting it so that it's longer on the top with fewer layers, with the bottom graduating into more layers. Oprah's hair grows quickly, and she's had shoulder-length hair, but she enjoys it most

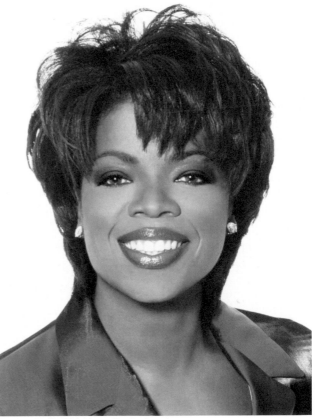

Skrebneski, © 1996, Harpo Productions, Inc.

when it's shorter. It's a fresher look for her, and she can easily handle it herself over the weekend without having to worry about it or have me style it for her.

This is a realization that Oprah has come to after years of playing with different styles. After all, hair should be fun. You might love the ease of short hair for years and years and suddenly wake up one morning tired of the same old thing. Or you might do as one long-haired friend of mine did after a scorching summer day: she marched right into a beauty salon and told the stylist, "Off!"—and loved the result so much that she kept her hair short for the next four years.

I'm not going to dictate which hairstyle you should get. I'm also not going to tell you *how* to cut your hair, since that's a job best left to a professional. If you try to take matters into your own hands without a beauty school diploma, you're asking for trouble.

Don't believe me? Check out Lila, an Italian-American with Type 3B corkscrews that she likes to wear blown-dry straight. Every six weeks or so, I shape her hair into a shoulder-length cut. I cut it with only a few long layers, so that gravity will weigh her curls down a bit; then I blow it out, and she leaves the salon looking great. And then six weeks later she returns with little pieces and short curls sticking up every which way. This is a routine that gets played out every time I see Lila. I ask her, "What happened here?" And every time she gives me this "Who me?" look and says, "I don't know what happened. I just cut a little bit out." Then I've got to repair the mess she's made. She does this again and again, not because she has a bad haircut but because she plays with her hair and doesn't take the time to blow-dry it properly (see Chapter 3 for blow-drying tips). So when it gets full and puffy, she hacks at it with scissors, thinking she can thin it out. All she really does, however, is make matters worse: the weight is gone from her hair, and the curls spring back up—exactly what she was trying to avoid. A lot of women do this, and it drives me nuts. I'm not trying to be a prima donna hairdresser, but it's extremely aggravating when you explain to people that they're ruining their haircut this way and then they pretend that they didn't do it. They always say, "What are you talking about? I just trimmed about a quarter of an inch because my hair was falling in my eyes." But in reality, three inches have disappeared mysteriously, and the women are not happy with what's left of their hair. So please, please, once you've found a perfect cut for you and your type, leave it alone. But first let me give you a few guidelines so you'll know what to look for before you get into that stylist's chair.

cutting it right

does your fine, thin Type 1 hair just lay about your shoulders, looking exhausted? Cut it off. Baby-soft Type 1 hair looks best cropped above the shoulders for more volume. A blunt-cut bob in an interesting geometric shape is my personal favorite for this hair type: it takes advantage of Type 1 shine and has drama and movement. Avoid cutting layers into your hair; they'll just make it look even thinner. The exception to that rule: a short, layered "boy" cut like Mia Farrow's in *Rosemary's Baby*.

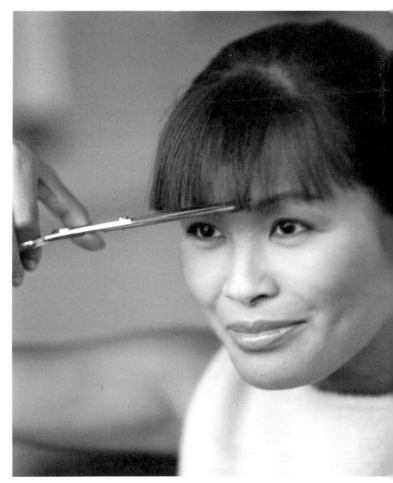

Toni Lynn Alford is a legal assistant and model with soft, fine, straight Type 1A hair. Toni's very athletic and loves this cut because it fits her personality. The layers around her face give the cut some sassy sex appeal, and it's long enough to pull back or pile up.

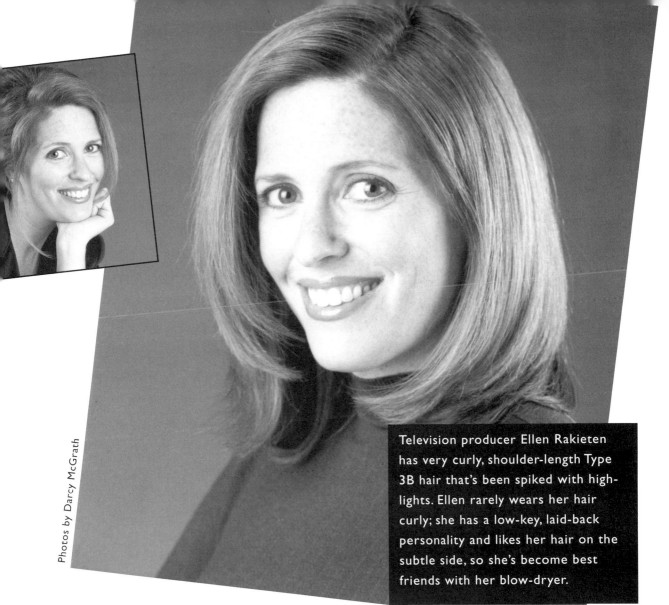

Photos by Darcy McGrath

Television producer Ellen Rakieten has very curly, shoulder-length Type 3B hair that's been spiked with highlights. Ellen rarely wears her hair curly; she has a low-key, laid-back personality and likes her hair on the subtle side, so she's become best friends with her blow-dryer.

Long Types 1B and 1C hair look great cut in soft layers that play up the face. The layers give a versatility that is a welcome relief from the basic long, straight, parted-down-the-middle style that makes so many women look like refugees from the sixties. Really thick, coarse, wiry hair works best with a little length in it. That way, you can control it more because it has some length to weigh it down. If it's too short, it tends to get very full and stand straight up. Of course, if you're into that look, that's great, too.

Wavy Type 2 hair works well in a variety of shapes and cuts, whether it's long, short or in between. Layers bring out the movement and texture in wavy hair, while blunt cuts tend to maintain a solid form. Still, layers will never add curl to the hair; short

Irene Michaels is a model, actress and journalist with long, wavy Type 2A hair. Irene absolutely loves long hair because it's feminine and versatile, and she can wear it braided, slicked back into a chignon or blow-dried straight for a contemporary look.

Photo by Darcy McGrath

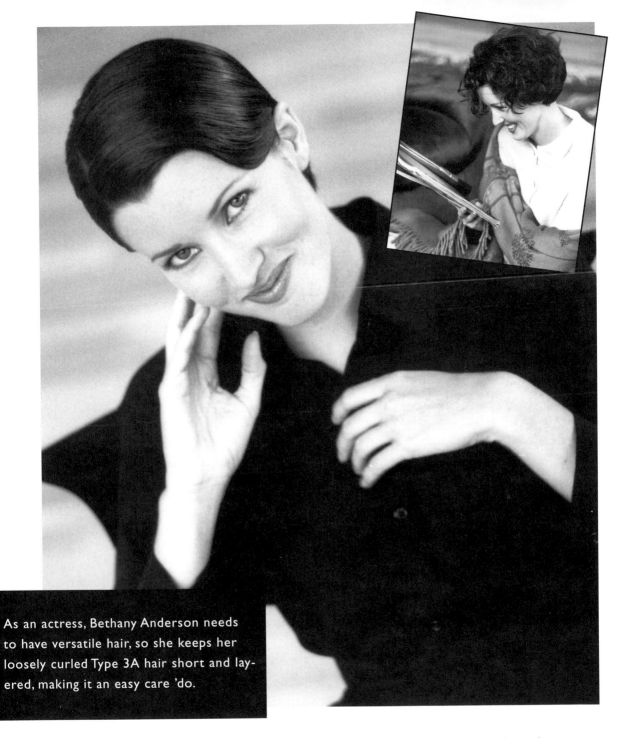

As an actress, Bethany Anderson needs to have versatile hair, so she keeps her loosely curled Type 3A hair short and layered, making it an easy care 'do.

wavy hair that's been layered will always look like short wavy hair that's been layered—unless, of course, you opt for a perm. But that's another story. Long blunt cuts are best on very coarse Type 2 hair; short layers will only add bulk and bushiness.

Curly Type 3 hair tends to be baby soft, which means it won't have a lot of weight to it. So if it's layered and not very long, it's going to get puffy—which Lila discovered every time she hacked at her hair with her scissors. This works great if you're going for a very short look or don't mind a round shape to your cut. Now, I don't mean that you can't layer longer curly hair, but it has to be done carefully so that it takes on more of an oval shape. I do this by paying painstaking attention and making sure that the top layers of the hair are longer than the ones on the bottom. Blunt cuts work best when the hair is longer, especially if you're going to dry it naturally. Again, you need weight to control those curls. If the hair is bobbed up to your neck, you're going to get that Rosanne Rosanna-Dana style (remember Gilda Radner's character from *Saturday Night Live*?), a look that was unattractive

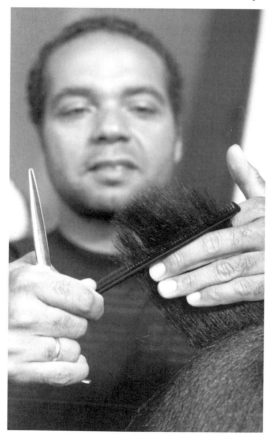

even in the 1970s.

When cutting curly hair, it's always a good idea to seek out someone who specializes in cutting Type 3 tresses. Why? The bends and twists of ringlets pose a unique haircutting challenge. For Type 3s, it's not unusual to walk out of a salon with an uneven mop of hair. I eliminate this problem by blow-drying the hair straight before cutting it—even if my client is going to wear her hair curly. That way, the curls aren't a distraction, and I can clearly see the lines of the hair. There are other stylists out there who believe that curly hair should only be cut wet. Whichever the case may be, find someone who knows what he's doing!

Cynthia Cabrera is a social worker who loves her naturally curly Type 3B hair— even though it sometimes has a personality of its own. Her hair is cut in one length, making it easier to control. And on days when it's doing its own thing, she can pile it up with ease.

Davida Rice is a super-busy entertainment attorney who puts in marathon hours at the office. Because she doesn't have time to fuss, she often keeps her long, healthy, relaxed Type 4A hair in a ponytail. This one-length cut provides her with a lot of styling options. It can be worn smooth and past her shoulders, or in a French twist.

Relaxed Type 4s should follow the same haircut guidelines as Type 1s; once you relax the hair, you've relaxed the texture out of it and can cut any shape into it. Still, relaxed hair left to its own devices will tend to frizz, so you're going to have to

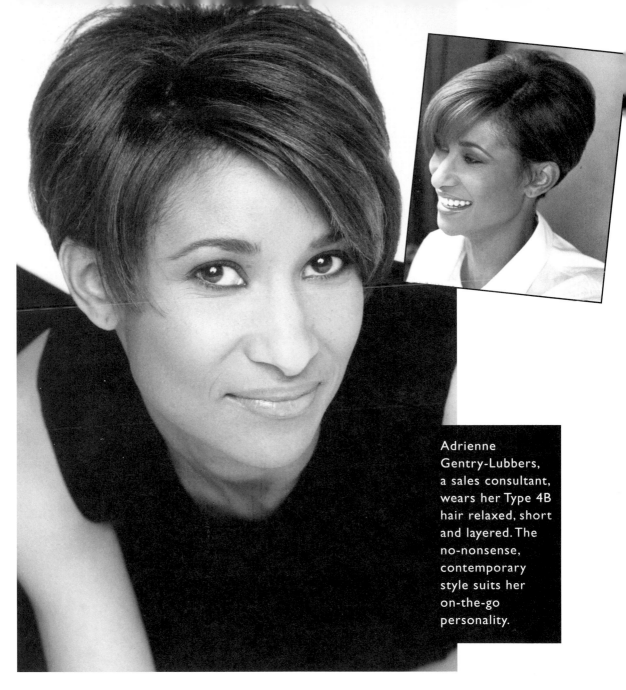

Adrienne Gentry-Lubbers, a sales consultant, wears her Type 4B hair relaxed, short and layered. The no-nonsense, contemporary style suits her on-the-go personality.

style it with a blow-dryer, rollers or a curling iron. Because they require the least amount of styling, bobs are probably the easiest cuts to handle. I love simple bobs blown dry straight; I think they look sophisticated and sleek. Short cuts almost always need to be layered; short blunt 'dos come off looking like helmet heads.

Natural Type 4s require totally different cutting techniques. While in its natural state, the most easy-care look out there is the TWA—teeny-weeny Afro—popularized by the model Roshumba and actress Cicely Tyson. You can wash it, let it air-dry and go. Big, fluffy Angela Davis 'fros are enjoying a renaissance, too. The style is cute—it looks modern, it looks good. But it takes a certain hair texture to give it that springy bubble effect like the Jackson Five and the Sylvers wore in the 1970s. Type 4Bs with a zigzag pattern will sprout giant-sized naturals that would do Michael Jackson proud, while Type 4As with tightly coiled hair will find that after washing their 'fro, it dries and shrinks. The natural needs a layered cut to release the kinks and coils of the hair. But to get the necessary length, you'll have to help things along by either braiding it wet until it dries (which can be time consuming), or blowing it out a bit with a blow-dryer (which can be damaging if you overdo it).

Now that you've got that perfect new 'do, it's time that you learn just what to do with it.

growing it out

You've had it with your short 'do and are longing for Rapunzel locks. What to do in the meantime? Whatever your hair texture, regular trims—every six to eight weeks—are a must to keep hair healthy. You only need to skim the ends to keep split ends under control. (Once an end splits, it doesn't stay put. Instead, it travels up the hair shaft, unraveling as it goes.) Regular trims not only keep split ends at bay, but they also keep the growing-out uglies away. How? Frequent mini-haircuts prune wayward locks into some sort of shape. If you're growing out a short, layered cut, for example, your stylist will keep trimming the longer bottom layers until the shorter upper layers of your cut catch up. Let's face it: growing out your hair from a very short cut to shoulder

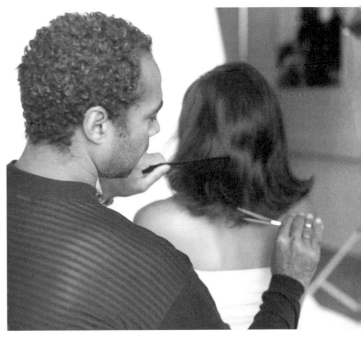

length requires patience—it can take anywhere from a year to eighteen months for Type 1s and Type 2s and eighteen months to two years for Type 3s and Type 4s—so you'll need all the help you can get to keep frustration at a minimum. You know what I'm talking about: unruly layers that, like Alfalfa's hair on *The Little Rascals*, stand straight up, saluting the air; cute little short cuts that suddenly turn into poodle 'dos; sleek TWAs that start doing a Buckwheat imitation. Hang in there through the rough spots and experiment with clips, barrettes and hats to disguise the most awkward growing-out stages. Another trick: slick wet hair back with a gel for a Josephine Baker look (Type 4s with natural hair may need to use a stocking cap until hair dries to keep it laying flat). Then cross your fingers and hope for the best. Growing your hair out is a waiting game.

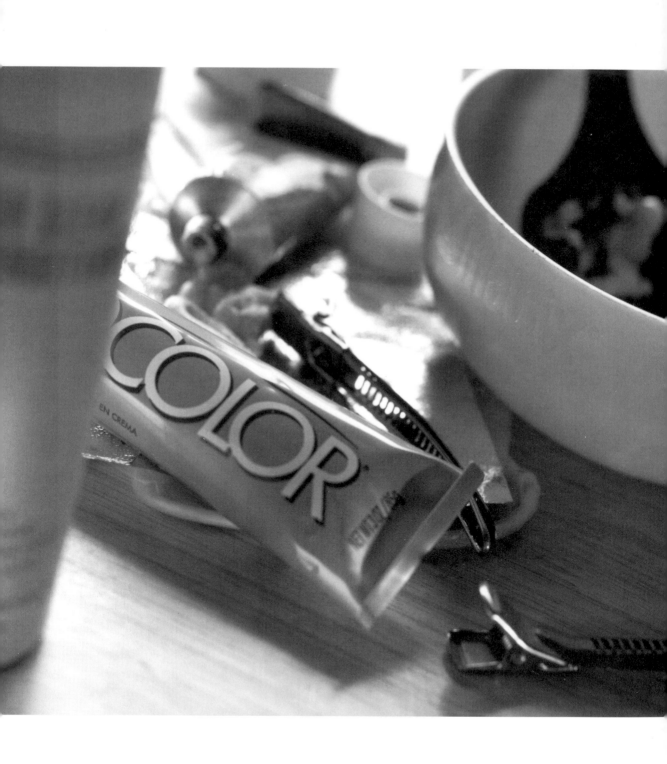

chapter five

messing
with
mother
nature

making the chemical connection work for you

There are two sides to the chemical story. Only the names have been changed—to protect the guilty *and* the innocent.

Take Tonya. If you asked her to describe her shoulder-length hair, she would tell you in no uncertain terms that her fine, thin Type 1 hair was like "seaweed on a rock." She hated it. It did nothing but cling to her head and straggle down to her shoulders. One day, I suggested that we try something new: since she was starting to gray—a fact that did not make Tonya happy—why not try coloring her hair? The hair color, a lovely strawberry-blond shade, covered her gray streaks. But better yet, it gave her hair some texture and much-needed volume, and it showed off her chic new bob. Tonya was thrilled with her bouncy new hair. No more seaweed.

And then there's Mia, who for years had been relaxing and coloring her Type 4 hair on a regular basis. Because we used only semipermanent color (more on that later) and religiously followed up with conditioning treatments, Mia's hair was healthy and strong. Until the day that my assistant, Bill, after relaxing her hair, mistakenly dumped a bowl of *permanent* color onto Mia's hair—and then put her under the dryer. The heat from the dryer baked the chemicals into Mia's hair, turning it bright orange—that's right, orange—right there on the spot. Mia freaked, and I rushed in to do emergency work. I colored her hair to cover the orange, tinting it a much darker shade than normal. Fortunately, Mia's hair didn't fall out, and the color turned out beautifully. But we still condition and color it regularly, waiting for the day that the ghastly orange shade underneath grows out for good. And, no, Bill doesn't work for me anymore.

As you can see from this tale of two chemicals, messing with Mother Nature isn't something to be taken lightly—unless, of course, you don't mind watching your hair break off in clumps or turn bizarre colors. Playing with chemicals is a tricky process. One false move and, at best, you're stuck with dry, damaged locks.

At worst, you're stuck with no hair—sometimes for good. But applied properly, chemicals—and by that I mean relaxers, permanent waves, curly perms, bleach, highlights, etc., etc.—can tame the most unruly mane and make it much easier to deal with. I'm not a back-to-nature freak; I'm all for doing whatever it takes to enhance the beauty God handed out at birth. I just believe that it should be done wisely. Most times, that means you can't combine chemical processes. Adding bleach and the like to permanent waves or relaxers is a disaster waiting to happen.

Let me give you an example. Early in my career, I met Carol, who straightened her Type 4 hair with a hot comb. (Type 4s tend to use chemical processes to control their hair more than any other type.) Carol was tired of the press-and-curl routine and was ready for a relaxer. No problem, right? Except that Carol had also highlighted her dark hair, and it was peppered with ugly brassy streaks. I warned her, "If you relax your hair, you're going to lose those streaks." She said, "That's fine, if it breaks off, it breaks off." So I relaxed her hair, and sure enough, as I rinsed the solution away, Carol's highlighted streaks literally melted away into a slimy goo that dissolved as it rinsed down the drain.

Fortunately for Carol, she had plenty of healthy hair left over. Her relaxer looked great and, better yet, no more brassy streaks. But that's not a risk I would ordinarily recommend anyone else taking. And whatever you do, don't try that trick at home! In fact, when it comes to chemical processes, I would discourage anyone from playing beauty parlor on herself. Go to a professional who's been trained to work with these processes. Many women try to save money and time by doing their own hair at home, but you'll end up spending *more* money to pay someone to undo what you did in the privacy of your own bathroom. Even if you're a professional, pay someone else to do your hair for you. It's difficult to see the back of your head; it's even harder to avoid processing already-processed hair again when you're trying to touch up the new growth. Trust me on this: damaging your hair is just not worth it.

Having said that, I will admit that it's not advisable to sit in the stylist's chair and blindly hand over all your faith and trust. There are stylists out there who will

"Oprah's hair is enormously flattering—up-to-date yet classic, chic yet sassy, easy to care for, functional and, above all, healthy."

sell you down the river, sacrificing your locks in favor of making a buck. A little education will protect you—and your hair. And guess what? That's what I'm here for. So read on for more about . . .

straightening it

ack in the post–World War II years, in an effort to be a hepcat, my dad used to "conk" his Type 4 hair. This was before the "black is beautiful" era, and at that time, fashionable African-American men all sported that conked look: smooth, gleaming, chemically straightened hair just like Nat King Cole's.

But if the look was smooth and easy, the method used to get it that way was quite the opposite: a foul, evil brew of Red Devil lye, potatoes, eggs and Vaseline that was combed through the hair. The concoction smelled awful—and stung even worse. The longer my dad could withstand the sting, the straighter his hair would be. To him, those monthly sessions in hair hell were well worth it: when he was done, my dad had a shiny, smooth head of slicker-than-slick waves.

We've come a long way since those primitive, fire-breathing chemical straighteners of the 1940s and 1950s. Technological advances have replaced the potatoes, eggs and Vaseline with sophisticated conditioners and milder chemicals. They no longer burn and leave the scalp a mass of scabs; instead of stripping the hair of life, the new relaxers leave the hair full of body. But they still *do* contain lye—or to be exact, sodium hydroxide, a chemical that straightens hair by breaking down the cuticle layers so that it lays flat. This is serious stuff. Once you apply this chemical to your hair, your hair is altered permanently. There's no turning back. The only way to return to your natural texture is to cut the treated hair off and start all over. (See "Growing It Out" at the end of this chapter for tips on easing out of a relaxer.)

But if you want to permanently straighten your hair, sodium hydroxide is the only way to go. Don't be fooled by relaxers that claim to be "no lye." Such claims are nothing more than clever marketing tools to get you to buy their product—a no-lye lie. "No-lye" relaxers are actually made of calcium hydroxide, which is just a milder form of lye. A "no-lye" relaxer functions by dissolving the hair cuticle, but since it's "milder," it doesn't break down the hair enough to flatten the cuticle layer and give some protection to the hair shaft. It actually leaves the hair shaft wide open to all sorts of damage. People who use "no-lye" relaxers have processed hair that looks dull and damaged; the hair can't reflect any light because the cuticles aren't lying flat and smooth. The result? No-shine hair. Over time, your hair will become more damaged using this type of relaxer. I don't like them and never use them. I also don't like the so-called conditioning relaxers or back-to-nature relaxers that purport to contain "natural" herbs. Believe me, an herb-enriched chemical is just another chemical.

Obviously, only certain Type 3s and most Type 4s are candidates for chemical straightening. If a curly Type 3 comes into my salon and wants her hair straightened, if it's at all possible, I try to talk her out of it. Instead, I teach her how to blow-dry her hair straight or wet-set it for the same effect. If it's too curly for that, then I will relax it. But even tight curls can be altered without chemicals; some Type 4s wanting straighter hair can do without chemicals as well. Relaxers will definitely dry out your hair, which means that you have to condition it more often. Relaxers require serious upkeep, so if you have curly or kinky hair, getting a relaxer won't be the answer to all your prayers. You'll still have to work with your hair, and, as Mia's story illustrates, you should forget about using a permanent hair color—unless you have superstrong hair that's kept very short so that the hair is always new. Two chemicals mixed together on textured hair like Type 3 and Type 4 is extremely damaging. Lots of people do it anyway, but they end up with hair that's very, very dry and very, very porous (when hair has been chemically damaged, the cuticle layers open, making the hair react like a sponge). Basically, their hair is way beyond repair, and it's not a pretty sight.

Type 3 curls can be relaxed, but remember that chemically straightened hair must be moisturized with conditioners often.

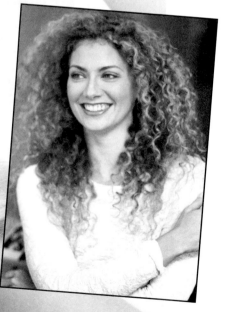

styling options

Going for a new look and you've absolutely got to have straight hair? Chemically relaxing Type 4 hair can give you styling ease to get the options you're looking for.

Having said that, I will admit that for many Type 4s, relaxers are the easiest way to take care of their hair. It makes combing the hair a relative breeze and provides a whole new array of hairstyling options. Hair that doesn't resist a comb raking through it is less likely to break. In its natural state, kinky hair (unless it's braided or dreadlocked) is hard to grow to great lengths because it's prone to snapping and breaking. The hair must be evenly relaxed so that it is one uniform texture: any difference in the degree of curl means that a comb will snag the hair and damage it. To prevent this, you need to maintain the consistency of your relaxer with regular touch-ups of the new growth. How often you need to do this will depend on your hair texture and how quickly your hair grows; usually it's every four to six weeks. I touch up Oprah's hair every five to six weeks.

Your hair texture will also determine whether you use a relaxer in mild, regular or extra-strength formulations. Most Type 4s will respond to the relaxer without a problem, but some who try to relax their hair find that it returns to its natural texture after the first shampoo. Why does this happen? Strong, healthy hair will resist the relaxing process; fine, curly hair will usually bounce right back because it is stronger, more elastic and more able to resist the breaking-down process. Hair that straightens easily is usually coarser, weaker hair. I can always tell at a glance which hair is going to relax and which hair is going to fight me. But if you've absolutely got to have straight hair, even the most resistant hair will eventually respond to relaxers. Sometimes the process has to be repeated again a week later. As you can imagine, this does damage the hair, but if done properly, it won't kill it.

keeping the spice alive

Maybe you love your kinks, curls and waves the way they are—you just wish they'd calm down a bit. In that case, you might want to consider texturizing the hair, a process in which the relaxer is combed through the hair (sometimes a little oil is added to the mixture) briefly to release some of the curl. This process works well on hair that has very tight corkscrews or hair that is coiled so tightly that, left in its natural state, it would contract, clinging closely to the head. (Type 4B hair, with a "Z" pattern, generally doesn't respond well to texturizing: the hair relaxes into frizz rather than curls.) This process can be done on long or short virgin hair; touching up new growth has to be done carefully so that the chemical doesn't overlap on already-processed hair, making it too straight and more susceptible to breakage. Successfully done, the relaxer will smooth the curls into a loose "S" pattern; the hair will look longer and softer. With a texturizer, many women are able to air-dry their hair for a "natural" look that shows off their springy curls. Of course, texturized hair can always be blown dry or wrap-set for a sleeker look.

Because straight hair is currently popular, there is a rash of new "anticurl" products out there that promise to smooth out curly and frizzy locks. Be careful: although many claim to "condition" the hair, they actually contain ammonium thioglycolate, which is the same chemical compound used in permanent-wave solutions. It's a much harsher chemical than lye relaxers, so I don't recommend these "anticurl" products at all. You can guarantee that they will dry your hair out, leaving it completely lifeless if you're not extremely careful. I also don't like the curly perms—Jheri curls, nouveau waves, dry curls, you name it—that were so popular in the 1980s. Talk about marketing madness. Print ads for these curly perms—and you know what I'm talking about—show models sporting bouncy, "carefree curls" that just need a spritz of so-and-so's miracle product to keep them looking fresh. The reality was, and still is, far from carefree. These perms contain ammonium thioglycolate and require a highly damaging two-step process: straightening the hair, rinsing it and then rolling it on rods and saturating it with even more solution. I won't do curly perms. I think they're highly unattractive, and if you indulge in them, instead of boasting a head full of curls, you'll be showing off a head full of Brillo. Never put chemical curls on top of relaxed hair—unless, of course, you're looking for an expensive way to go bald.

Keep your
kinks, curls and
waves *and* have
manageability
by texturizing.

curling it

for all you Type 1s out there with fine, droopy locks, I can sympathize. It's frustrating dealing with a mane that has no body or shape, trying to handle hair that laughs at your best efforts to puff it up. So you try to force the issue, saturating your hair with gels, lotions and sprays—only to be left with hair that looks and feels like a motorcycle helmet. Then you fry it with curling irons and electric rollers and—*voilà!*—you create something that *looks* like a curl. But it collapses in defeat at the slightest sign of humidity. In desperation, you run to your friendly neighborhood beauty parlor, where you plunk down no small sum to have curls put in permanently. Then you're left with a 'do that would make even the Bride of Frankenstein cringe. And now you're stuck in a rut, investing hundreds upon hundreds of dollars to keep your head full of chemical curls. Because while your perm might look goofy, it looks truly scary when it starts to grow out and you're left with two-toned hair that's flat on top and freaked out on the bottom.

Sound familiar? We all want what we don't have. But before you plunk down your cash on a permanent wave, proceed cautiously. I have to admit, I'm biased. I don't like them. I can't help it, but whenever I think of permanent waves I think of frizzed-out mall hair that has no shape and looks as if it's been electrocuted. To me, it's a highly unattractive style.

Now that I've gotten that off my chest, let me explain how permanent waves work. Like relaxers, permanent waves restructure the hair. Permanently. Once you put them in your hair, that's what you're stuck with. During the process, Type 1 hair (and sometimes Type 2 and even loosely curled Type 3) is shampooed and then rolled on rods or rollers. (The choice depends on the amount of curl you're after. The larger the rod, the bigger, or looser, the curl.) The rolled hair is then saturated with ammonium thioglycolate. The hair then takes on whatever shape it's been rolled into. Those so-called root perms that curl the roots of the hair for volume are a waste of time. They add just a little texture to the hair and leave a big mess: hair that kinks at the scalp and has straight, flyaway ends.

Even though I dislike perms, I must admit that they're good if you've got stick-straight hair and feel you absolutely must have a curly look that's going to last. But remember, you're putting chemicals into your hair. Perms will dry hair out, and if they're not applied properly and the chemicals are left on too long, you'll be left with overprocessed, frizzy locks. To prevent this, don't perm color-treated hair (perming bleached hair is asking for hair drama), and go to a professional who knows what he or she is doing.

But to me, it's not worth it. Perms are such an old-fashioned approach to styling Type 1 hair. I love straight hair when it's got a great cut and has been styled for maximum volume. I feel so strongly about this that whenever someone comes into my salon begging for a perm, I strongly discourage them. If they insist, I refer them to someone else in the salon. A final note: sometimes Type 3s with ultracurly locks are advised to get curly perms to reset their curls in a looser pattern. I don't recommend this method either.

coloring it

not so long ago, coloring your hair was a top-secret activity kept deeeeep in the closet. If they did it at all, good girls kept quiet about it; only bad girls let the world know what was up with their bleached-out hair and blacker-than-black roots. Remember the ads that asked, "Does she or doesn't she? Only her hairdresser knows for sure"? Fortunately, times have changed, and hair-coloring has come out of the closet in a big way. Everyone, it seems, is doing it. Supermodels like Linda Evangelista brag about their rapid-fire color changes; television commercials show women doing it themselves in some very public places, from buses to their own weddings. OK, so maybe they're overstating the point just a bit. Still, it's high time women had some fun with their hair color.

And why not? I'm a big fan of hair color. A good coloring job can add shine, polish, highlights, warmth, drama and fun to your hair. It can also cover gray, tame wild hair and pump up "seaweed on a rock" locks like Tonya's, making the hair easier to blow-dry and style. American women love to color their hair. Statistics show that about 90 percent of women in this country play with hair color in one form or another. The majority do it to cover gray; younger women experiment with highlights; others still go for the shock effect of hyperbleached hair or two-toned "skunk" streaks.

Despite the current craze for crazy color, a good color job should look as natural as possible, like the subtle richness that you see in the hair of a very young child. Look for colors that occur naturally: auburn reds, strawberry blonds, sandy blonds, warm chestnuts and glossy ebony shades. Nature never intended for us to have burgundy, pitch-black or fire-engine red hair. Whichever process you decide to go with—if you decide to play at all—educate yourself before you subject your hair to your colorful whims. Mistakes are hard to correct. And trust me, a lot of those supermodels and actresses sporting multiple color jobs might look wonderful in photos, but if you looked at their hair up close and personal, you'd be shocked at the damage. A lot of them end up reviving the very short haircut out of necessity. Which brings me to another point: make sure your hair is in tip-top condition before you color it. If it's damaged before you put chemicals in it, it's only going to look that much worse afterward.

doing it permanently or just till it washes out

Basically, there are two types of hair color: permanent and semipermanent. Semipermanent color coats the hair and washes out over time; permanent color breaks down the hair cuticle and deposits pigment into the hair shaft. Semipermanent color covers gray temporarily and can only darken hair; permanent color covers gray more extensively and can lighten hair as well. Even so, it's best to stay within two shades of your natural color, even when using permanent color. Dark-haired women who try to go lighter without bleaching it first with peroxide end up with that ghastly, orange hair. Again, if your hair is relaxed or permed, you can only use semipermanent rinses—unless you want to see your hair melt in the shower, just like Mia.

Semipermanent rinses or glazes look great on Type 3s and 4s; they add shine and give the hair a plastic coating that tames frizz and enhances your natural color. The darker the color, the more shine you'll get. Textured hair tends to be dry, and light hair colors can make the hair look woolly.

bleaching it

Marilyn Monroe did it and launched her career. Today, a lot of younger women in the spotlight are taking her lead and playing with bleached-out locks—for instance, the actresses Ashley Judd, Mira Sorvino, Geena Davis and Marisa Tomei. It's not an easy look to accomplish; if your skin is olive or dark, it looks very unnatural. Bleaching also is quite rough on dark hair, since it involves a two-step process: the natural color is stripped with peroxide, then the hair is dyed the desired shade of blond with a permanent hair color.

At one time, African-American women (those who weren't born that way) who bleached their hair were considered to be the ultimate in tacky. Now, some consider them the ultimate in hip—look at up-and-coming acting talent Jada Pinkett. My assistant wears her cropped, natural hair bleached a funky platinum shade. I think it looks fabulous because it flatters her honey-brown skin. But she's young, and believe me, youth is essential to pull this look off; it can look quite harsh on older women.

Because the process is so damaging, fragile Type 4s—and some Type 3s—are better off wearing their bleached hair short, natural and unstraightened. This way, the hair is kept so short that the damaged parts are trimmed off constantly. After the process, the hair is so fragile that you can't blow-dry it or style it with curling irons and the like. The bleach might actually straighten the hair a bit, so a spiky, short cut is the easiest way to go with this look. Do anything more to it, and your hair is almost guaranteed to fall out.

h i g h l i g h t s

Highlights are small streaks of color scattered throughout the hair for a flattering effect. Usually, it is done in a one-step process, using permanent color to lighten parts of your natural hair color by a few shades. Any type hair can be highlighted, although brunettes should stick to reddish, rather than blond, highlights. Type 2s in particular look great highlighted—the lighter color brightens the hair, jazzing up the wave pattern for a spectacular effect. Type 3 hair needs thicker highlights so that the streaks don't get lost in the curls; relaxed Type 4 hair can be highlighted only if it is kept very short.

h e n n a

Henna was outrageously popular in the 1970s, touted as a "natural" hair color. But I don't recommend it. Made of plants and herbs, henna works by literally baking the color into your hair. It jams the cuticle with herbs that won't wash away—they have to be cut out. Colorists that I work with describe henna as a "curse," because its effects never go away. Because it's made of natural ingredients, you can't control the results you're going to get from it. In fact, henna-treated hair won't take to a perm at all. It does make the hair extremely shiny, but it gives your locks a false sense of security; henna-treated hair actually loses elasticity and, when stressed, can snap right off.

d o i n g   i t   a t   h o m e

Don't. Color-treated hair always looks better in the hands of experts. Most processes are too complicated to try at home with any hope for good results; it's also really difficult to touch up the roots. Even the most rudimentary procedures— for instance, lightweight highlighting and semipermanent color rinses—look better when done in a salon. A good professional can help you pick out colors that will

coloring it

truly flatter your skin tones: the hair color shown on the box won't be the color that you see on your hair when all is said and done. Also, at-home products just aren't as effective; most semipermanent rinses that you can buy in a drugstore will wash out in about a week.

Still, I know that many of you don't have the time or the money to invest in costly and time-consuming trips to the salon. So if you're going to take your hair into your own hands, be extremely careful. Follow the directions to the letter. And leave the heavy-duty jobs to us.

one more thing

Sometimes you have to break the rules. Sometimes you have to use something to damage your hair to make it more manageable or just more attractive. Just be smart when you do it.

rapid-fire red
growing it out

Tired of living your life enslaved to chemicals and frequent trips to the beauty parlor? The good news: there is life outside the world of peroxide and sodium hydroxide. The bad news: it's going to take a lot of patience to get there.

More and more women are opting for a more natural approach to their hair, turning away from chemical relaxers or permanent waves. Others are learning to love every single strand of their gray tresses—without the aid of Clairol No. 5.

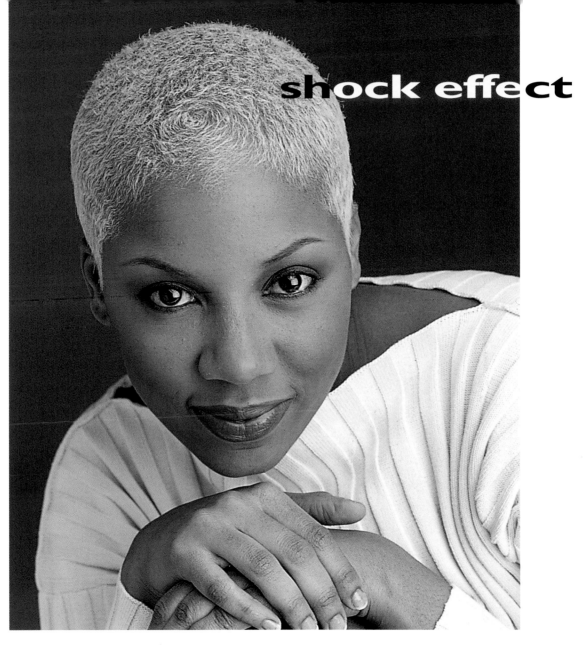

shock effect

Generally speaking, chemical-free hair is healthier hair; it's also a lot less expensive to maintain. So how do you get there when you don't even remember what your natural hair texture or color really looks like? Well, if you're relaxing it or curling it with permanent-wave solutions, the path of least resistance is the most radical route: cut it all off. No, I'm not talking about shaving your head; I'm saying wait until you have several inches of new growth—this should take about three months

color has come out of the closet in a big way

or so—before snipping off the chemically treated portion of your hair. This way you can start fresh with a head full of healthy, virgin hair. Think of it as a clean start. This all-or-nothing approach is also the healthiest for your hair. Why? As your hair grows out, you will have two radically different textures of hair on your head. If the new growth is kinky and the old hair is straight as a board, as you comb your hair, the comb will snag as it tries to make its way through the two-toned morass of hair. What happens then? Snap. Your hair is breaking off in the comb. The same thing happens with curly-permed hair, although to a lesser degree, because the difference in textures between straight and wavy/curly hair isn't as extreme.

So what do you do if you can't bear to part with your hair in such a dramatic move? Proceed with caution. Curly-permed hair should be blow-dried straight to minimize the difference in textures, until it has completely grown out. Trim away a half inch or so of the permed hair every month until the untreated hair catches up to the desired length. And condition, condition, condition.

Growing out relaxed hair takes a little more patience and care. Wear hairstyles that disguise your two-toned texture (braids or twists) or set your hair for a curly look. Be very careful when combing your hair: always use a detangling conditioner when you comb it after a shampoo. Opt for wet sets and wrap sets over blow-drying and curling irons, and whatever you do, don't press the new growth straight with a hot comb. You're just asking for trouble. You should always treat

"I'm a big fan of hair color. A good coloring job can add shine, polish, highlights, warmth, drama and fun to your hair."

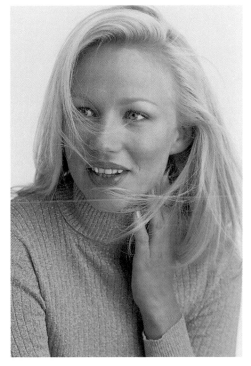

your hair like it's your most prized possession, but during this growing-out time, be extra tender. Deep-condition regularly and spend the night luxuriating on satin pillows—they'll treat your hair with kindness.

Ready to return to your natural hair color? If it's been permanently colored or bleached, again, chopping your hair to the roots is the easiest option. Or you can endure the bicolored look—in some fashionable circles, dark roots on blond hair is the ultimate in

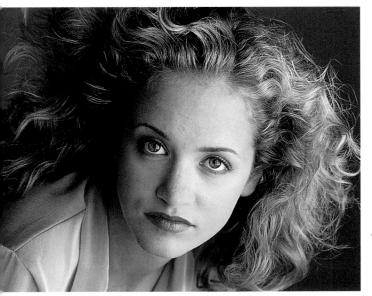

chic. Or you can use a semipermanent rinse in a color closest to your natural shade on top of the permanent color until your hair has grown out completely.

"Type 2s look great highlighted— the lighter color brightens the hair, jazzing up the wave pattern for a spectacular effect."

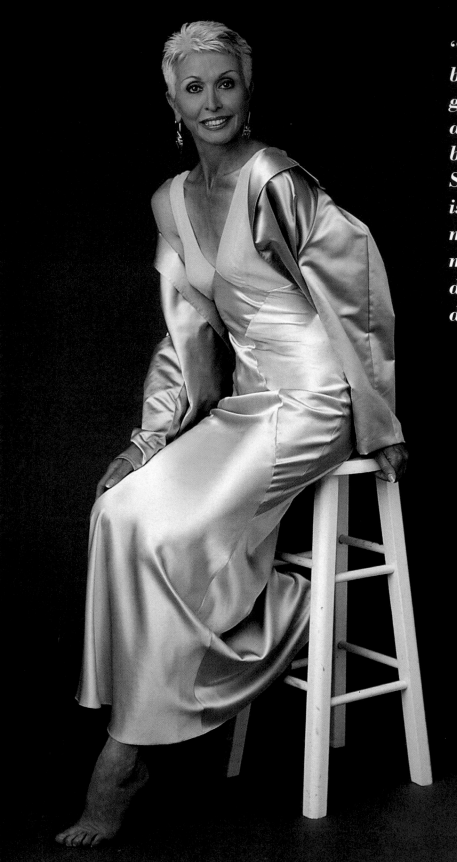

"I've come to believe that gray hair like age (to quote baseball great Satchel Paige) is an issue of mind over matter: if you don't mind, it doesn't matter."

silver
is gold

photographed by
Darcy McGrath

attitude is everything

"Sure, gray hair isn't for everyone—it takes a certain amount of panache to pull it off. But if silver tresses flatter you, then why not leave well enough alone?"

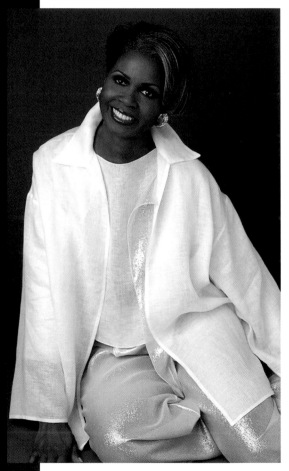

caring for gray hair—even if it's hiding under a layer of no. 5 auburn gold

I have a confession to make: I have a thing, a serious thing, for gray hair. Maybe it's because my mother has gray hair—and of course, she lets only me do her hair—but a well-cut, healthy head of silver hair does it for me every time. Silver locks look sophisticated, mature, regal. Think of Bill Cosby's lovely wife, Camille, with her sharp, closely cropped natural. Or the model Carmen, an ageless beauty who always looks perfectly coiffed with her shoulder-length pageboy.

Still, I have to admit that I didn't always feel this way about gray hair. In fact, it took my mother to turn me around. A few years ago, when those white streaks first started popping up, I suggested that she color her hair. I thought it made her look older, and I didn't want my mother looking old. My mother is a very pretty lady who's very comfortable with herself, and she didn't give her gray hair a second thought. She was perfectly fine with it, but she went through with the coloring because she knew that it made me happy. What can I say? She's my mom. When it comes to her hair, she basically lets me do whatever I want to do to it; I don't have to convince her to try something new. She let me know that it wasn't necessary for me to cover her gray, but if I wanted to do it, then I should do it.

So I colored her curly hair a very pretty reddish-brown shade. It looked great— at least I thought so—and I thought it took years off of her. But soon, I could tell that she wasn't happy with it. She would complain about the texture (coloring does tend to dry the hair) and about having to touch it up; she hated all the upkeep that it required. But she never once said, "I don't like this red hair. It just isn't me." When I finally took the hint, and cut off the tinted hair, she was very happy. Today she wears her silver hair extremely short, and I think she's beautiful. And now I realize that it was me who needed to change, not my mom. It wasn't that she looked old; I was the one who felt old—and I was projecting that onto her. Without saying anything, my mother taught me a valuable lesson about self-acceptance.

Of course, I wasn't alone in my antigray bias. Most people associate gray hair with age, yanking out those white strands just as fast as they crop up. But I've come

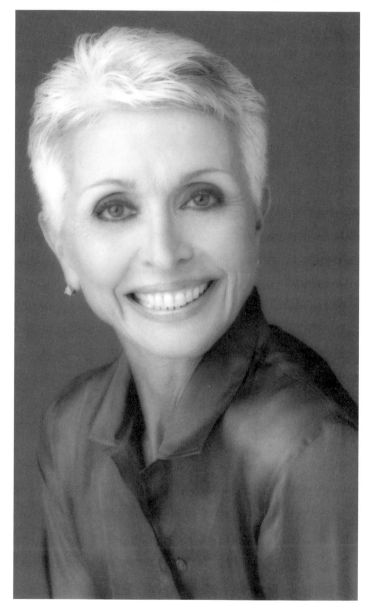

to believe that gray hair is like what baseball great Satchel Paige said about aging: it's an issue of mind over matter, because if you don't mind, it doesn't matter. If you feel like you look older with gray hair, then you project that. If you're in shape, your face looks great and you have a fabulous haircut, you can look ageless. Sure, gray hair isn't for everyone—it takes a certain amount of panache, not to mention the right skin tone, to pull it off. But if silver tresses flatter you, then why not leave well enough alone?

Now don't get me wrong, having gray hair poses its own unique set of problems. Regardless of whether you decide to go au naturel or cover up with a layer of No. 5 auburn gold, gray hair isn't ordinary hair. Anyone who's old enough—and in many cases, young enough—to find that snowy stuff sprouting on her head knows that it is more wiry than pigmented hair. It's usually drier, coarser and appears to have a life of its own. The rest of your hair may lay down meekly, but gray hair has a way of standing at attention and yelling, "Here I am!"

Why? First of all, gray hair is hair that has completely lost its pigmentation. This is a gradual process; the hair shaft loses pigment until it is completely white. Gray hair is usually hereditary, although some premature graying is associated with certain medical disorders. Take a look at your parents, and you'll get a pretty clear picture of where you're headed. Most folks spot their first strands when they hit their late thirties; others get premature sprinkles in their early twenties or even as young as age twelve. Others don't gray until quite late in life, if at all.

When your hair grays, the nutrients that give it its color are gone. The result? Completely color-free hair. The amount of gray hair you have depends on what your hair will look like: hair that is pure white is hair that is 100 percent gray; if your hair looks like salt and pepper mixed together, then roughly 50 percent of your hair is actually gray. Hair that looks like it has a silver cast to it is usually about 75 percent gray, with 25 percent of the natural color remaining. As much as I now love gray hair, I like it the least when it's in the early stages—a few sprinkles here and there up to about 25 percent. To me it

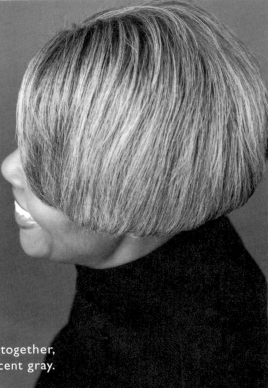

If your hair looks like salt and pepper mixed together,
then you are actually 50 percent gray.

"Today she wears her silver hair extremely short and I think she's beautiful."

looks mousy. I think it is best then to cover the gray with a rinse until the unpigmented hair catches up to the rest of the hair for that salt-and-pepper look. (Refer to Chapter 5 for more on coloring your hair.)

I first started coloring Oprah's hair with a semipermanent rinse to give it some shine every time I relaxed her hair. About a year ago, I noticed that she was starting to get a few gray sprinkles scattered through her hair. Now we use the semipermanent rinse to give her hair shine *and* to cover the gray; the tint is a fairly light color, so it just gives her gray strands a highlighted look and her hair a certain sparkle. Which is fine with Oprah—she's not at all fond of those gray streaks. When the rinse starts to fade and the streaks start popping up again, she always says, "Oh, my gray hair is coming out, let's cover it." But from my experience with my mother, I've learned to gray and let gray, so whatever she wants is fine with me.

Generally, the darker the hair, the more graceful the graying process. Lighter hair—from light brown to red and blond—usually looks dirty until it is completely gray. If you're not interested in completely covering the gray, it's best to add highlights to the entire head until the gray grows in completely. The highlights add dimension to your hair and blend in the gray.

care and feeding

n the early 1990s, I was asked to style then–First Lady Barbara Bush's hair for her appearance on Oprah's show to promote *Millie's Book*. I was excited, but my excitement was soon replaced with anxiety—not at the prospect of styling the first lady's hair, but by the major-league security check the Secret Service did on me before I was allowed to stand within ten feet of her. I had nightmare visions, imagining that somewhere out there, Big Brother was keeping tabs on every little thing I did (not that I have anything to hide). Once I met Mrs. Bush, however, I was more at ease. I found her to be very friendly, very warm and extremely easy to work with. She wasn't the sort of first lady to travel with a hairstylist, so she was open to whatever I suggested.

Still, because Mrs. Bush's beautiful snowy hair has always been her trademark, I didn't want to change her look too much. Besides, her deeply wavy Type 2 hair was already nicely shaped from a recent cut by her personal stylist, so she didn't need much work. In fact, her hair was a testimony to the beauty of wearing gray au naturel: it was well maintained, damage-free and a pure white color. After I shampooed her hair, I blew it dry, being careful to keep the blow-dryer moving so that I didn't singe her hair. (Burned gray hair looks fried and turns colors. I didn't want to be the stylist responsible for leaving scorch marks on the first lady's hair.) I finished things off with a cool curling iron, and that was it. She was happy, and as far as I know, I'm still in good standing with Big Brother.

Mrs. Bush's hair is a "Do," a perfect example of what you should do if you choose to let your gray show. *Do* take meticulous care of it, because whatever you *do* to it, it will show. Because gray hair often acts like a sponge, it can change colors, looking ashy or dingy, depending on what you put on your hair or into your body. You probably already know that swimming in a chlorinated pool can turn your hair a weird shade that nature never intended. But did you know that if your hair is gray and you drink orange juice (or eat anything containing citrus) a day or two before getting a relaxer, you can end up with acid-yellow hair?

A little prevention and common sense is all that it takes to keep your snowy hair looking great—of course, the prescription depends on your hair type. If you're a Type 1 and have an oily scalp, you'll need to shampoo daily. Your regular shampoo is fine for everyday, but it's a good idea to substitute it once a week or so with a "bluing" shampoo. These shampoos, specially formulated for gray hair, contain bluing agents similar to what your mother used on clothes to make them whiter. Like those laundry detergents, the bluing shampoos prevent hair from taking on a yellowish tinge. Every two weeks or so, use a light cream rinse to keep hair manageable; use a deep conditioner once a month to keep hair in tip-top shape. If you're a Type 1 with fine hair, you'll be glad to know that gray hair will give you some much-needed body and texture. Be careful using gels and hairsprays to style your hair. Gels that are clear or blue are fine. Again, with any other colored gel, your hair will absorb the color—which is fine if you want candy-colored locks.

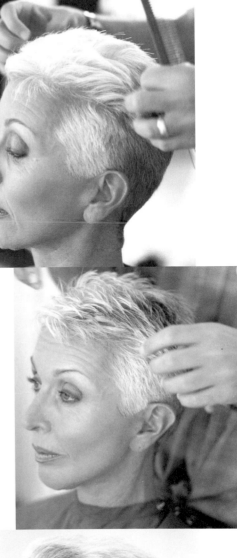

Geometric cuts beautifully play up both the texture and color of Type 1 hair. Gray hair serves as an exclamation point for a really precise hair cut. So don't ruin your hair with permanent waves and the like. It's just not necessary, and you could end up frying your hair in the process.

Type 2 hair doesn't require such frequent shampooing; a good sudsing every other day should do the trick. Type 2 hair will benefit from an occasional cream rinse. Deep-condition twice a month and be careful with heat appliances like curling irons, blow-dryers and hot rollers. Again, heat can scorch your hair. Trust me—toasted gray hair looks and smells burned. Gray Type 2 hair looks best when its waves are kept above the shoulders. When it's longer, the waves just become overpowering.

Type 3 hair becomes more resistant to styling as it grays. The wiry strands tend to stick out and defy your best efforts to keep it under control; sometimes the curl pattern of the hair even changes as it grays. It can even become straighter and lose some of its elasticity, almost always becoming more coarse and more dry.

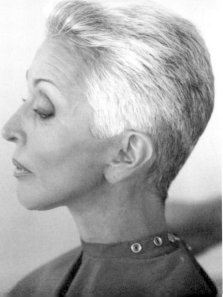

To keep Type 3 hair manageable, you'll need to shampoo it every other day or so with a moisturizing shampoo. Always follow up with a conditioning rinse to tame unruly locks and invest in alcohol-free mousses and gels. Once Type 3 hair has progressed to the salt-and-pepper stage, *cut it off.* Curly gray hair should be kept cut above the shoulders, or even shorter. I see women sporting gray Type 3 that hangs out around their shoulder blades, thinking they look absolutely fabulous. Now, I applaud anyone who feels that good about herself. And while I believe that these women have a right to be proud of their beautiful gray—after all, they earned it—I think that long, naturally curly gray hair is very, very unattractive. Its sheer volume tends to overwhelm the face, making the wearer look hard, much older and witchlike. If you've just got to have long hair, then straighten it, either with a blow-dryer or a relaxer. Personally, I love a styled, straight look. It just seems prettier to me, unless you keep your hair very short and curly—like my mom!—which can be very attractive also.

Case in point: Elise, a Jewish woman with long, bouncy curls that fell way below her shoulders in back and were cut in short bangs in the front. At the time, her hair was 50 percent gray. There was so much of it that when you saw her coming, the first thing you thought was, "Look at that mass of gray hair." You couldn't see how pretty she was. I talked her into shortening her hair, shaping it into more of a layered cut to blend all the hair lengths together and wearing it straight. After she agreed—making it very clear that she didn't want to go short—I turned her mane into a smooth, layered shaggy style; the blow-drying straightened things out so that her hair wasn't the first thing you saw about her. Sure, you noticed Elise's gray hair, but it was pretty and soft. And it took years off of her lovely face.

Like Type 3s, Type 4 hair requires conditioning every time it is shampooed. Gray hair that's been relaxed is more prone to discoloration, so you'll need to use a bluing shampoo to maintain your white hair color. Weekly deep-conditioning treatments are a must. Remember, Type 4 hair is more fragile than other types. But while it may be more delicate, silver Type 4 hair looks great in a variety of ways. Short, naturally kinky Type 4 hair looks wonderful. Long hair works well for gray

Type 4s, too. In fact, when you have kinky gray hair, you have a lot of styling options, although blunt cuts are almost always easier to manage. I like graying Type 4s best in a nice bob that's been straightened.

But however you decide to wear your gray hair, whether you're a Type 4 or a Type 1 or somewhere in between, wear it with pride. Remember, it's all about mind over matter. Take care of your hair, keep your makeup, dress and attitude up-to-date, and you're sure to turn heads.

"Geometric cuts beautifully play up both the texture and color of salt and pepper hair."

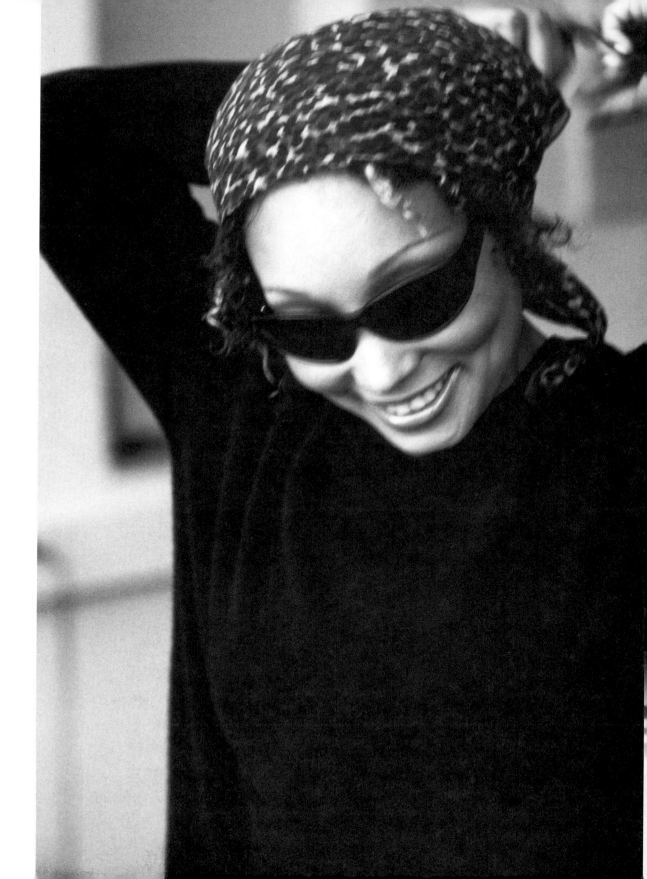

chapter seven

damage control

how to handle the hairy curveballs life can throw your way

Twenty years ago, Alice came to me with a mystery. She'd always taken her Type 3 hair for granted. It was thick, healthy, shiny, soft, chemical-free and full of supertight little corkscrew curls that she straightened with a blow-dryer. Now, however, it was coming out in handfuls. In fact, it seemed that her entire head was being taken over by large, gaping bald spots—some of them as large as a silver dollar. As you can imagine, she was terribly upset; she didn't know what was happening. Could I help her?

Well, I took one look at Alice's hair and knew that her problem was greater than anything that a hairdresser's tools could handle. I like to think of myself as a hair doctor, but clearly, I was out of my league here. Remember, Alice's hair—what was left of it—was strong and free of chemicals. There were no broken chunks of hair, no ragged split ends, no evidence of foul play to the scalp. So I knew that her hair loss couldn't be blamed on woman-inflicted damage from relaxers, color treatments, blow-dryers, hot combs or curling irons. There was nothing that I could do, beyond putting her on a regimen of scalp-stimulating shampoos and conditioners to keep the rest of her hair healthy. I urged her to see a dermatologist—right away.

The dermatologist diagnosed Alice's condition as alopecia areata, a medical condition that results in abnormal hair loss (more on that in just a bit), and prescribed a course of medication. In a few months, Alice's hair was back in full force, once again growing healthy and thick. From time to time, the bald spots would return, but it was nothing that we couldn't handle. There was no need for Alice to freak out; she and I both knew exactly what to do.

Happy ending? Not quite. You see, a few years ago, Alice, then in her early fifties, discovered that she had breast cancer. Fortunately, the cancer was arrested in time, but the recovery proved to be long and painful. After undergoing a radical mastectomy, like most cancer survivors, Alice went through a series of debilitating chemotherapy treatments. Once again, she started losing her hair. But this time, the hair loss that she suffered made her previous alopecia look like child's play: she was almost completely bald. Over the years, we'd become friends, and I was so worried about her. Luckily, Alice is a very strong woman and was able to make sense of it all; she accepted what she had to do to make things better. And in this case, there was little she *could* do; until the chemotherapy was finished, she would continue to lose her hair at a rapid pace. All I could do was crop her remaining hair close to her scalp and tell her about her options: wigs or scarves. Alice opted for a good-looking wig while she waited things out. In time, Alice regained her health—and her hair. From her, I learned a valuable lesson about maintaining grace and good humor in the most trying of situations.

Alice's health problems would challenge the strongest of women. Losing your hair is a frightening thing under any circumstances; losing your hair as a result of cancer or any other life-threatening illness can be overwhelming, shaking the soul to its core. Of course, if you're fighting for your life, whether you've got hair while you're waging war is of secondary importance. But I believe that if you feel good about how you look—and consequently, feel better about yourself—it can go a long way in speeding up the healing process. This is true whether you've got a mild case of alopecia, you find that after the baby your hair isn't what it used to be, or you're struggling with cancer. But first, in order to feel better, you've got to know what to do.

To help you figure things out, I've called on the expertise of my friend, Dr. Jonith Breadon, a well-respected Chicago dermatologist. We both agree that most of the problems discussed in this chapter require a doctor's intervention. Sometimes, a seemingly minor hair problem can be an indication of a much more serious medical condition. So please, please, please, *see a doctor right away.*

alopecia

Suddenly, your thicker-than-thick hair is thinner than thin. Or, like Alice, you're suddenly noticing huge bald spots scattered throughout your head. Or you've been using a hot comb for years and literally have cooked your hair into oblivion. Or maybe, as you get older, you're starting to look more and more like your father—especially when it comes to his disappearing hair.

Many men will spend a fortune seeking out magic potions that promise to return their scalp to its former glory—or even just return a few hairs. Men lose their hair. They don't like it, but most accept it as a fact of life, part and parcel of the inevitable aging process. For women, however, losing their hair carries with it a certain amount of shame; going bald just isn't considered feminine. The fact is, one-third of all women will grapple with hair loss at some point in time. Fortunately, it's usually not permanent. With a little medical help, most problems can easily be solved.

Thinning hair, female-pattern baldness and sudden hair loss are all different versions of alopecia. "Alopecia" is a fairly generic medical term; it can be caused by a variety of factors, ranging from genetics to infections to serious diseases. Alopecia areata, the condition Alice suffers from, is actually a fairly rare immune disorder that usually occurs in the young (children can get it when they're babies; it's unusual to see it occur for the first time in anyone over forty). This form of alopecia occurs because the immune system has kicked into high gear; overactive white blood cells attack the hair follicles as if they were the enemy—as if they were a virus or some other infection. The result: damaged hair follicles. The hair falls out; sometimes total baldness results. Usually, women first become aware of the problem when they discover a shiny bald spot—and usually, they don't remember losing their hair. Although the condition is medical, for women in their twenties it is stress related.

The good news: with alopecia areata, the hair spontaneously grows back within six months. Like Alice, most will suffer with repeated bouts, but the overall prognosis is quite good for adults; children are far more likely to suffer permanent hair loss.

Female-pattern baldness (androgenic alopecia) is a fact of life; many women will find their hair thinning to an alarming degree as they age. We all shed about a hundred or so hairs daily; since we average about 100,000 hairs on our head at any given time, this is no big deal. In fact, you've got to lose more than 60 percent of your hair before others start noticing any appreciable difference. So, usually, your hair loss is never as extreme as you think it is. Most women who experience female-pattern baldness can point to a balding male member of the family who passed his hair genes along to them. The good news is that, unlike men, who frequently suffer from a receding hairline, women will maintain their hairline. So the term "female-pattern baldness" is actually something of a misnomer. Don't worry. You'll never go completely bald; your hair will just get very, very thin. But we can solve that, too.

To be sure, alopecia is annoying, but in most cases it poses no real threat to your overall health. Sometimes, however, it is a sign of much more serious problems. If your hair loss is accompanied by excess facial and body hair (hirsutism) and severe acne, then you may have a tumor on your ovary that's producing too much of the male hormones testosterone or androgen. See your gynecologist right away. Other illnesses, such as hypothyroidism, lupus or syphilis, can cause serious hair loss as well.

Then there is the hair loss that you inflict upon yourself. Traumatic alopecia is caused by harsh chemicals—permanent waves, relaxers, curly perms, overenthusiastic bleaching—or overly aggressive styling habits such as tighter-than-tight braids, sleeping in rollers and wearing skinned-back ponytails over the years. With chemical abuse, the hair will eventually return, but repeated tension on any part of the scalp causes scar tissue to form. What happens then? The hair follicle is replaced by scar tissue. Which means no more hair. Ever. You won't see the effects right away, but after fifteen years of overzealous hair yanking, you will. It makes me sad to see a woman with bald spots on either side of her head from years of wearing slick ponytails as a kid. Then you take a look at her young daughter with a thick head of hair, wearing the same hairstyle, and you know history is going to repeat itself. Traumatic alopecia is always a preventable hair loss.

Hot-comb alopecia is seen in women who have used a hot comb since they were children to straighten their hair. In this case, the baldness is usually seen at the crown of the head, because it happens when the extreme heat of the comb melts the oils used to lubricate the hair. The burning oils drip into the scalp, causing folliculitis, or infection of the hair follicles, which eventually damages the scalp to the point that the hair follicles are destroyed permanently.

treating it

There are different treatments available for the different types of alopecia. With alopecia areata, your doctor will first try to calm down your immune system, injecting the area with cortisone shots every three to four weeks until the regrowth appears. The success rate with this treatment is quite high: more than 60 percent. If that doesn't work, your doctor then may try anthralin, a derivative of anthracite coal, which works to sensitize the area so that the immune cells stop attacking the hair follicles. Another method is using the drug dinitrochlorobenzene, which works in the same way. Neither method is as successful as cortisone. If you've suffered complete hair loss, cortisone might be injected or taken orally. With either of these methods, you're more susceptible to not-so-nice side effects like weight gain, water retention, high blood pressure and elevated blood sugar levels. Another treatment for complete hair loss is PUVA—the drug Psoralen plus UVA light treatment. A solution is applied to the affected area, and then the area is exposed to a light box. Again, this treatment works by suppressing the immune system; the success rate is less than 50 percent.

With female-pattern baldness, the drug minoxidil (known commercially as Rogaine) can solve the problem to a large degree. In fact, women respond better to Rogaine than most men do. The drug is applied topically, and you'll see either a cessation in hair loss or new hair growing back. This new growth ranges from normal textured adult (or "terminal") hair to finer "baby" (or velus) hair—or both. The new growth will cover the baldness, but chances are, you won't have luxuriously thick hair again. Also, taking minoxidil is a life-long proposition: as soon as you stop taking it, the new growth will fall out. A possible side effect is increased facial hair.

For most trauma-related hair loss from excessive chemicals, such as bleach, relaxers and hair dyes, the cure is simple: stop it. Because the hair shaft is weakened but not permanently damaged, the hair almost always grows back. So lay off the chemicals until new hair grows in. And next time, treat your precious hair a little more kindly.

If your hair loss results from infections of the hair follicle, antibiotics will clear things up quickly. Fungus infections such as ringworm, which is found mostly in children, are treated with daily medication taken orally. Syphilis requires a penicillin injection.

heavy medication

lassic cancer-fighting treatments like chemotherapy affect hair that is in its growth phase. Because 90 percent of all scalp hair is in this phase at one time, hair loss from these drugs is quite extensive. As Alice found out, there is nothing you can do during this time except to wait it out. These days, there are a variety of attractive wigs, hats and scarves that you can wear to get you through this difficult period. Look for support groups and special programs like "Look Good . . . Feel Better" (call 1–800–395–LOOK), which gives women cancer survivors makeovers, in your area.

Some non-cancer-fighting drugs, from heavy dosages of vitamin A to arthritis medications, tend to affect scalp hair that is in its shedding phase, accelerating the shedding process. Because this affects only 10 percent of your hair, the hair loss won't be as noticeable to others. (Remember, others won't take notice until you've lost more than half your normal hair.) The only remedy is to stop taking the drug. Ask your doctor to find a substitute.

Repeated radiation therapy usually won't affect your hair, unless you have a brain tumor or skin cancer and the area being radiated is your scalp. This course of treatment is designed to kill tumors in their active growth phase; it also kills anything with a high cell turnover, such as hair. Consequently, radiation could cause some hair loss and permanent scarring, but it's not likely to result in total baldness.

The constant barrage of drugs to fight opportunistic illnesses means that AIDS sufferers may lose their hair. Some will find that their hair changes texture, growing in lighter in color and finer in texture; others will find their hair prematurely grays at an accelerated rate, sometimes turning completely white. Unfortunately, until researchers find a cure, nothing can be done.

dandruff or dry scalp?

Your scalp is on fire; a snowstorm of white flakes floats down from it, settling on your shoulders in an unsightly mess. You scratch the itch, dust off the flakes, saturate your scalp with hot-oil treatments. Nothing changes. What to do? Is it just a dry scalp, or is it dandruff, described in television commercials as a guaranteed killer of social lives?

The answer? None of the above. Both the itchy scalp and nasty white flakes are actually the by-products of an all-too-common skin condition called seborrheic dermatitis, or increased production of skin cells. Many of us will do battle with flare-ups of sebborhea at some point; stress and seasonal changes—like extremely cold winters—tend to bring it on. You don't have to have "dandruff" flakes to have sebborhea; many folks plagued by it just complain of that old bugaboo: dry, itchy scalp. It's a mistake to try to solve the problem by oiling the scalp; all the moisturizers, hair ointments and conditioning treatments in the world won't ease the itch.

treating it

Instead, look for over-the-counter dandruff shampoos that contain either zinc pyrithione, tar or salicylic acid. Tar will cut down the increased cell turnover rate so that the skin cells stop growing so quickly, flaking off in embarrassing chunks. Zinc kills fungus and yeast (some experts theorize that's the cause of sebborhea); salicylic acid works by exfoliating the excess dead skin cells. Pick a shampoo specially formulated for your hair type.

These over-the-counter shampoos should be used daily; most folks will see dramatic improvement within the first week. After that, follow up with a weekly treatment to keep the itch and flakes at bay. If your hair is relaxed, ask your dermatologist to prescribe a cortisone-based cream that you can apply directly to the scalp. (Itchy scalp sufferers might find more relief from this ointment as well.) Should the problem persist, see your doctor for stepped-up treatments. Sebborhea is a condition that is never really cured, but it can certainly be controlled.

Sometimes, those white flakes that you see don't have anything to do with sebborhea—you're just overdoing it with the styling products. How can you tell? With sebborhea, if you look closely, you can see the flakes actually lifting away from the scalp; product buildup flakes off from the individual strands of hair. Excessive flaking—and I do mean excessive—is sometimes a symptom of the HIV virus. When in doubt, always see a doctor.

eczema

eczema is a skin condition that results in an unattractive, itchy rash. Usually, it is confined to the body, but eczema can and does crop up on the scalp. Eczema won't cause hair loss, but its nagging itch can start a vicious itch/scratch cycle that can lead to hair breakage from the constant rubbing. When confronted with eczema, your best bet is to seek medical attention right away. The sooner you treat it, the better you'll feel. Again, cortisone creams work wonders, and again, this is a condition that can only be controlled, not cured.

pregnancy

Jane, a woman in her late thirties, loved being pregnant. Her hair grew thicker and faster than ever before, bouncing in thick waves down the middle of her back. It seemed sturdier than ever: nothing that she did to it, it seemed, could harm her hair. Highlights? No problem. Blow-dryers? No sweat. Under the heady influence of hormones, her hair thrived. Until the baby was born. Suddenly, her hair just wasn't what it used to be. It was dry. It was brittle. It refused to grow. Even worse, it was shedding like crazy. Highlights? Big problem. Her hair started to snap, crackle and pop. Blow-dryers? Just added insult to injury. Jane put up with the aggravation for nine months. Then she got pregnant again, and her hair sprang back to life. It grew, it grooved, and she was loving it. Then the baby was born, and two months later the same nightmare started all over again. Being a doctor, Jane understood what was happening; she knew she had to wait it out. It didn't make things any easier; Jane was depressed. She missed her big hair. Now, whenever she blow-dried her hair, it looked like stringy little rat tails. She chopped off her hair and brushed what

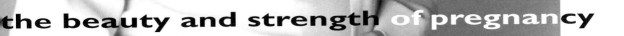

the beauty and strength of pregnancy

healthy, pure, natural

was left, counting the months until this hormone blowout ceased. Eventually, her hair grew back. But it never returned to her pregnancy glory days.

Of course Jane's hair wouldn't be the same as it was when she was pregnant. During pregnancy, your entire body is in overdrive; everything works better and more efficiently. After your baby is born, estrogen levels in your body abruptly drop. The result? Some women experience excessive hair shedding of up to 30 percent; the hair may also become hard to handle. Like Jane, you have to be patient when this happens and wait it out—usually the same amount of time it took you to conceive and give birth. Minoxidil, while safe for pregnant women and nursing mothers, is a waste of time: by the time the minoxidil kicks in, the hormones will have stabilized and your hair will be back to its prepregnancy self. In the meantime, be kind to yourself and treat your hair and scalp to a regimen of tender loving care with protein moisturizing shampoos and conditioners.

nutrition and your hair

Let there be no doubt about it: there are no miracle pills, powders or potions that can make your hair grow thicker or faster. Eating wonder foods or popping prenatal vitamins when you're not pregnant won't make your hair more abundant. Of course, you should eat a healthy diet rich in vitamins and minerals, proteins, green leafy vegetables and fresh fruits and drink plenty of water. Crash diets and marathon fasts can result in iron deficiencies that can lead to hair loss. Eating disorders such as anorexia nervosa or bulimia do affect the condition of your hair. Many sufferers find that their hair will become more sparse, finer in texture and will change color, usually to a reddish shade if your hair is dark. Once you resume eating normally, the hair returns to normal.

one more thing

Do take your health seriously. If you notice any sudden changes in the condition of your hair, see a doctor. Remember, if you take care of your health, your hair will take care of you.

nutrition and your hair

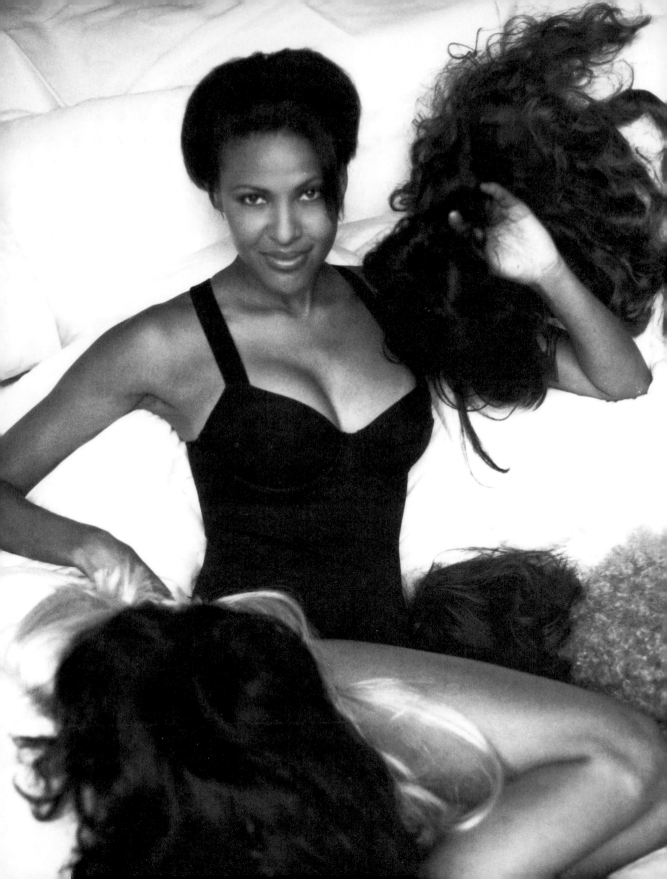

chapter eight

gilding
the lily

expanding on what mother nature handed out

Extensions. Wigs. Weaves. Wiglets. Hairpieces. Falls. Mother's Little Helpers. R&B crooner Alexander O'Neal bashed them in his hit song from the late 1980s, "Fake." And you remember how in the film *I'm Gonna Git You Sucka* Keenen Ivory Wayans smacked his lips, all ready for romance with Ms. Right, until, with a flip of a wig, she turned into Ms. Wrong. That is, Ms. Wrong with a bald pate and one teeny-tiny curl, smack dab in the middle of her forehead. From television sitcoms to Eddie Murphy's movies to the corner barbershop, nothing gets a laugh faster than cracking a joke about some wannabe sporting fake hair. Admit it. Maybe you've cracked a few yourself.

The jokes might be funny—OK, I admit it, I've laughed, too—but I don't think they're fair. Think about it. In ancient Egypt, with Cleopatra and her pals, elaborate wigs were all the rage. In other parts of Africa, from B.C. to A.D., women used whatever it took—wool, leaves, cotton—to add length to their beautiful braids. On these shores during the Revolutionary War, men and women alike wore animal hair powdered white and piled high atop their heads, often leaving a cloud of dust in their wake.

Let's face it. We've been helping out Mother Nature since time began. We're still doing it—except that now we've got an attitude about it. Piling on some store-bought hair is seen as a cop-out, the last province of the pretentious. But as I see it, there's nothing wrong with gilding the lily—in moderation. Maybe you want to experiment with a new look. Maybe you want to give your hair a rest. Maybe your hair is thinning and you want to give it a little extra oomph. Maybe you like flinging hair over your shoulders every once in a while. Why not? Go for it.

You'll be in good company. Celebrities like Oprah, Robin Givens, Tina Turner, Whitney Houston, Roseanne, Bo Derek and Patti LaBelle have all experimented with synthetic tresses. In fact, these days, women of all races and all types are demanding hair that's long, longer, longest and thick, thicker, thickest. It doesn't mean that they're trying to be something they're not. They just like having options. Weaves are coming out of the closet. When Oprah showed off her shoulder-length pageboy on her show, she had no problem telling the world, "This is a weave!"

Don't get me wrong. I'm not saying everyone should rush right out and invest in someone else's hair. I just think that, like a hairbrush or a blow-dryer, weaves, wigs and extensions can be useful styling tools. A little artificial hair can let you try on a new look. If your hair is fragile, wearing a weave can protect it for awhile. It can give your crop some much-needed volume. But like anything else in life, too much of a good thing amounts to abuse. And trust me, a lot of folks abuse wigs and weaves.

What do I mean by abuse? Some people think that getting a weave or a wig is the answer to all their questions. They don't do what it takes to keep them looking good. We've all seen those women wearing weaves that look like an animal with a severe case of mange. Or those church ladies who have been hiding under helmet-like wigs for so long that no one remembers what their hair looks like. Or those heavy metal rock stars with extensions so long that even Mother Nature is getting a good laugh at their expense.

If you're going to fake it, you've got to do it right. And doing it right means, above all, making sure that your natural hair is kept clean, conditioned and stress-free. So before you reach for that plug of hair, make sure that you do your homework. Read on, and I'll tell you everything you need to know about . . .

wigs and hairpieces

y mother was one of those ladies in the 1960s and 1970s who wore those curly wiglets. She used to send them out to be cleaned and styled—until, that is, I decided that I could do them myself. At the time, I didn't take it too seriously. It was just something for me to play with. I enjoyed

fashion

can be easily achieved with a funky up-'do and that little black dress, but when your hair is too short to pile up, a hairpiece or wiglet styled with your natural hair is the perfect enhancer.

making my mom look good, and she enjoyed it, too. She didn't want me going to beauty school, but she sure did want me styling her wigs.

Working with my mother's hairpieces, I learned that if you're looking for a change without making a commitment, you can't beat wigs, wiglets, falls, hairpieces and pin-on ponytails. Put one on, and in an instant you've got a new look. If you have long hair, you can have short hair for a day—and vice versa. You can go from being a blonde to a brunette or a redhead or even someone with a Day-Glo 'fro. It's a fun thing to do, and it can give your hair a much-needed break.

These little enhancers come in a variety of shapes, sizes, lengths and colors. You can buy either human hair or synthetic. Personally, I prefer human hair be-

cause you can style it yourself, but if you're all thumbs, synthetic hair is an easier choice. The style is built in, even after you wash it. (If you really want to change the style, see the end of this chapter.)

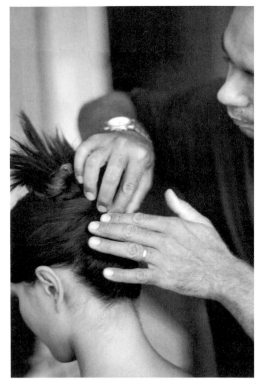

If you're wearing a hairpiece and some or all of your natural hair will show, please, please, please make sure that the color and texture of your piece match your natural hair—unless, of course, you're deliberately trying to achieve a mismatched look. The exception, of course, is wefts of loose hair that are pinned into your hair. You can pin in blond highlights or even colors like shocking pink for a fun effect. When *Essence* was planning a cover shot of Oprah, they wanted me to highlight her hair for a different look. As I said earlier, I don't like highlights on relaxed hair. In order to fake it, I took pieces of medium golden-blond hair and pinned it through Oprah's hair. It mixed with her chestnut brown hair for a really nice effect. After the shoot was over, she went out,

sophistication

goes hand in hand with formal, but
if you want to make a statement,
put aside the classic French
twist and add a pin-on ponytail
to your God-given tresses for a
more creative up-'do.

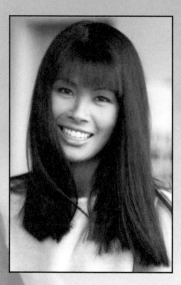

fun

is the key word here. Put one on and you've got an instant new look. Brunette to blonde, short to long, you can't beat wigs, falls and hairpieces for giving you change without commitment.

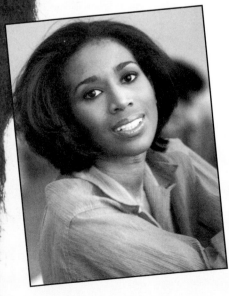

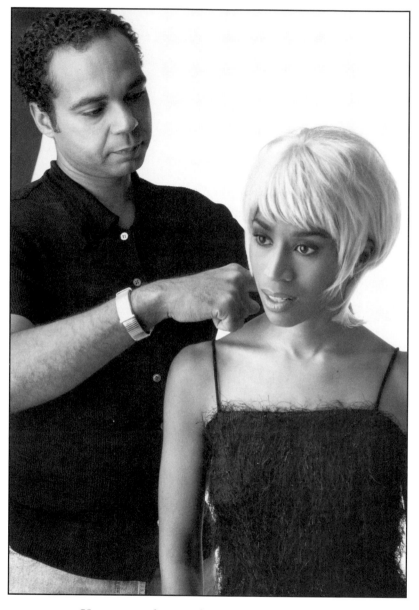

You can end up with severe scalp problems—and no hair at all.

enjoyed the highlights. The next day, when she combed her hair, she took them out.

Fun is a key word here. You don't want to make your wigs and hairpieces a permanent extension of your head. I don't recommend wearing them all the time, unless you have a condition like alopecia or you've lost your hair through chemotherapy and you absolutely must wear one (see Chapter 7 for more on this subject). In particular, wearing a wig puts a lot of tension on your hairline because the hair is always pressed under the wig. Time and time again, I see women whose natural hair is very damaged and broken from constant wig use. It doesn't stop there.

care and feeding

Synthetic hair is the easiest to care for. Wash it in your bathroom sink with a mild detergent like Woolite, rinse it, shake it out, let it dry on a wig stand and you're good to go. Human hair, on the other hand, requires a little more work. If it's a wig, send it to a salon specializing in wig styling, where they will set it, blow it, condition it and treat it as if it were your own hair.

extensions and weaves

from time to time, Oprah likes to take a little break from the daily styling—and from me. She usually picks a hair type that she can wash and wear, and a weave specialist puts the hair in. Before this happens, she and I discuss how we're going to style the weave, how long it should be and so forth. Since we want her to look as natural as possible, we agree that we'll cut it above her shoulders. This way she can give her hair a break and enjoy not having to think about it during her vacation months. Sounds easy, right?

Except that when the weaver puts in the hair, and the woven hair is hanging down Oprah's back, something takes over her. She becomes a different woman; there's this total metamorphosis, from the way she looks at herself in the mirror to the way she plays with her new hair and flings it over her shoulders. She becomes this character with all this hair—and suddenly she can't bear to part with her hair. It's happened twice, and each time she told me, "We have to think about this haircut. I don't think I want it too short." So even though we agreed in advance how I would cut and style her hair, now I have to cut it in three stages. It's the only time I fight with her. Every time I snip a little piece, she freaks out. It's as if she spent her whole life growing her hair and I'm trying to cut her bald.

But Oprah's not the only one. I see this happen to a lot of women, no matter what their race or how long their own hair may be. In an instant, they've got these long flowing tresses, and they're like, "I want to keep it; this is mine." There's something very seductive about instantly acquiring a massive mane; it can make you feel like Miss Glamorous or become a security blanket.

Still, when Oprah does indulge in a weave, it's always in the spirit of fun, regardless of how much of a personality change she may temporarily undergo. She does it at a time when she's not going to be photographed much, and for a brief period it does make life easier for her. We always pick Italian hair that has a slightly wavy texture to it. After the weave is in place, Oprah can shampoo it, put styling gel on it, let it dry and she's gone. She can work out in it; she can swim in it. If she really wants it coiffed, it's easy for her to go to a salon in a hotel on the road and trust someone to style it, rather than having to haul me around.

She loves that it gives her different hair—not to mention a different hair color—to play with, and that's fun. She doesn't care what people think about the weave, letting them know in no uncertain terms that it *is* a weave. When she takes it out after two months, her natural hair looks and feels strong and healthy. I think she looks great—with or without a weave. I recommend weaves for a change of style, not for perpetrating a fraud. I hear people say, "You should see my hair underneath this weave, it's really grown." If it's really grown, why not take off the weave? Let down your hair for awhile. You've got to come out from under your weave at some point. Why would you want to pretend it's your own hair?

A lot of people think that getting a weave or hair extensions will make their hair grow. That's a myth. At best, they'll give your hair a break for a maximum of eight to twelve weeks, period. Your hair needs proper conditioning and shampooing. If it doesn't get the nutrients that it needs, then it starts to dry out and break off. So if you wear your weave any longer than the recommended time, you'll have hair that looks worse than it did before you started playing with synthetics. I see some supermodels (no names!) who have made million-dollar careers out of wearing

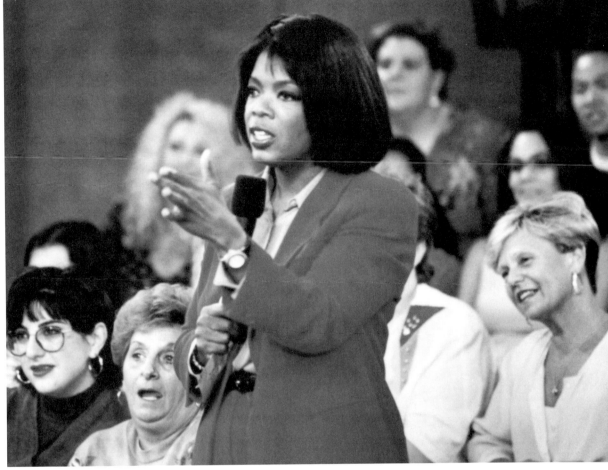

Steve Green, © 1995, Harpo Productions, Inc.

weaves. You never see their natural hair. And no wonder. Take a closer look around their hairline. You'll notice that their own hair has worn so thin that they literally *have* to wear a weave.

Enough lecturing. You get the picture. As I said earlier, take care of your hair, and it'll take care of you. One way to guarantee this is to seek out a good professional who knows what she's doing. Go to a salon that just does weaves. In other words, like Oprah, go to a specialist. If you break your leg, you don't go to an eye doctor, do you? The same holds true for your hair. Someone who does one thing all the time generally has made all the mistakes that are going to be made—before you ever walk through her door. Find someone who understands weaves, someone who knows how to style and cut them. Ask around, stop people on the street whose weaves you admire. But whatever you do, don't try this at home! You won't be happy with the results.

You should also know exactly the type of weave you want. The terms "weave" and "hair extensions" are used interchangeably, but they're not the same thing. With hair extensions, plugs of hair are braided into the natural hair. The hair can then be braided from the scalp to the ends or just braided and attached to the scalp with the rest of the hair left to hang free. Whitney Houston usually uses this method, as do Robin Givens and Janet Jackson. This method is great if you want a curly look or if you want your hair to really move. With this look, you can part the hair anywhere you want to part it. Generally, hair extensions don't work as well with straight hair because it doesn't hide the braids as well.

With weaves, a weft of hair (a row of hair stitched together) is woven through the hair. You can use weaves in just one section of your hair or all over your head. In either case, weaves can be done one of two ways: through bonding, where the weft is glued to the scalp row by row, or by sewing the weft onto a row of cornrowed hair. I don't recommend hair bonding at all. It comes loose too quickly, and I don't like the idea of applying glue to the very tender skin of your scalp. Some stylists bond the hair to the scalp; others glue it to the root of the hair. With bonding, it's difficult to comb your own hair, and you have to use additional chemicals to re-move the glue when you take out the weave. Everyone I've seen with bonded hair falls into the Bad Weave category. Plus, when the wind blows, tousling your hair, everyone can see your glued-on tracks. Tacky, tacky, tacky. Bonded hair is indeed cheaper and quicker than sewn-in weaves, but you'll be sorry in the long run.

Sewn-in weaves are a kinder, gentler option. With this method, your hair is first braided into tiny cornrows; the hairline is left free to blend in later with the woven hair. The stylist then takes a weft and sews it into an individual cornrow; the num-ber of wefts used is determined by the desired thickness. This can be a time-consuming affair—from three to eight hours—but I think it's worth every minute.

glamour

seems to be a given after you instantly acquire a massive mane with hair-weaves or extensions. You'll be in good company— many celebrities have experimented with synthetic tresses. And if you like throwing your hair over your shoulders every once in a while, then why not go for it?

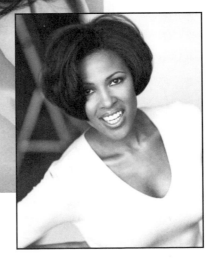

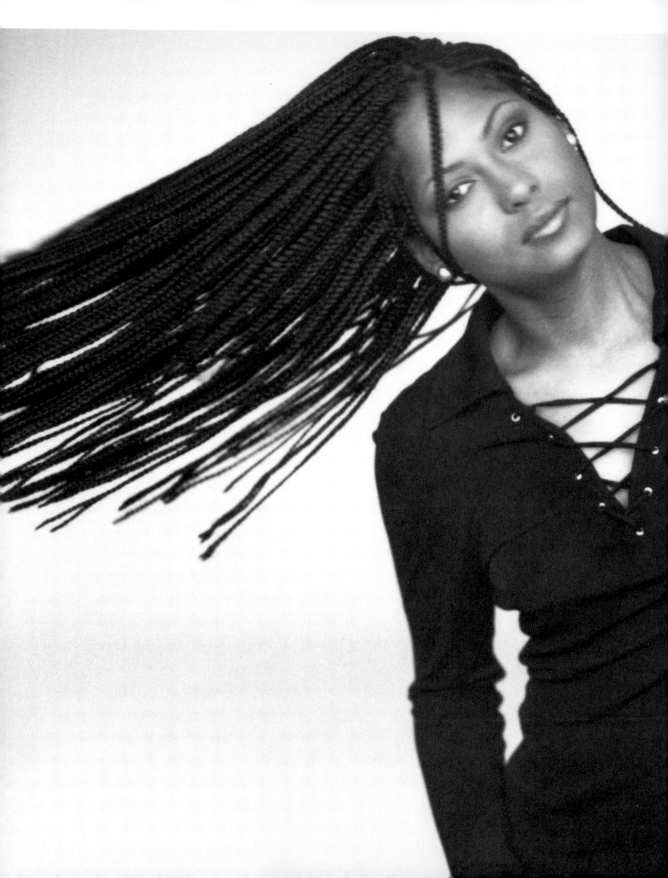

fake or for real

Picking a method is easy compared with picking what kind of hair you want lying next to yours. Again, quality is key. There are dozens of different hair types from which to choose, from synthetic to human to animal (that's right, usually yak, a kinky-haired ox). Synthetic hair is good for braiding. In the past, it looked fake—very vinyl and overly shiny—but technology has improved so much that synthetic hair looks just as good as the real thing. You can buy it in a range of textures from stick straight to kinky.

I much prefer human hair, but remember, not all hair is created alike. Some human hair on the market has been chemically processed (usually color-treated or permanently waved) so much that it's damaged before you ever put it on your head. My favorite hair to work with is "French Refined." The name is misleading (usually the hair is from either Asian or Mediterranean women); it just means that the hair is high quality and hasn't been processed. Again, like synthetic, you can find it in a variety of textures, including "Imported Afro Hair."

care and feeding

Not everyone likes weaves. In a Los Angeles pre-interview with comic Ellen DeGeneres, Oprah was wearing a weave. Ellen complimented her on her new 'do, and Oprah said, "Oh, girl, this is a weave." Ellen freaked: "Oprah, don't tell me you have a weave. There's no telling what's in there under your weave. They attract all kinds of things in there." Ha, ha. Very funny. But turnabout is fair play. When Ellen came to Chicago to tape the show, we had a little surprise for her: a videotape showing me cutting Oprah's weave out. In the video, every time I dug my hands into Oprah's weave, I pulled something out. "Wow," I'd say, pulling out an appliance that no male likes to be without, "so *that's* where my remote control went." Next it was my keys: "I've been looking *everywhere* for these." We had the last laugh.

As Oprah's little joke on Ellen illustrates, taking care of your weave is crucial to the health of your hair—not that strange objects will be magically drawn to your weave! Wearing a weave doesn't mean that your life will be completely carefree. First, you've got to find someone who knows how to cut weaves. This isn't necessarily the person who just put it in. So many times, I see women who have spent a ton of money on their weaves but haven't followed through with a really nice cut. A good haircut looks polished—you do want to show off your new 'do, don't you?

As your hair grows, the weave will loosen, so you'll need to have it tightened every six weeks or so. Synthetic hair is the easiest to care for, requiring nothing more than a shampoo, while human hair can be treated like your own. You can use lotions, gels, mousses, pomades and hairspray to style it. If you have braided extensions, braid experts recommend that you shampoo your hair while wearing a stocking cap to keep the braids intact. If you have a weave, be very careful not to pull on the cornrows during a shampoo. Putting excess stress on the hair will loosen the weave.

Like your own hair, French Refined needs tender loving care to keep it healthy. So by all means, if you want a straight look, buy straight hair and vice versa. Don't buy curly hair and then waste your time and money trying to straighten it. This is supposed to make your life easier, not more difficult.

one more thing

Whether you opt for hair extensions or a weave, it can be an expensive proposition. Hair is sold by weight. Again, the better the quality of hair, the more it's going to cost you. Synthetic hair can be as low as $10 a package (you'll need at least 5 packages), with human hair running you as high as $200 for a quarter pound. Once you've purchased the hair, it can cost you anywhere from a couple hundred dollars to thousands to have it put in. (The average cost is around $500 to $600 for a full head.) If someone offers to do your full head for $100, run. Trust me: you get what you pay for.

changing the texture
of your wig or hairpiece

f you're particularly handy, you can change the texture of your synthetic hairpiece. If your wiglet is curly and you're hankering for a smooth look, all you need is an electric clothing steamer to literally steam the curl out. Hang your hairpiece over your hand, and run the steamer up and down until the wave is steamed out. Steam the hair as you'd steam the wrinkles out of a pair of pants. Want to put curls into your straight wig? Section off a piece of hair and run the steamer over it until it is warm and damp but not wet. Roll the hair up in a roller and pin it. Move on to the next section until the entire wig is done. Then take the steamer and run it over all the rollers.

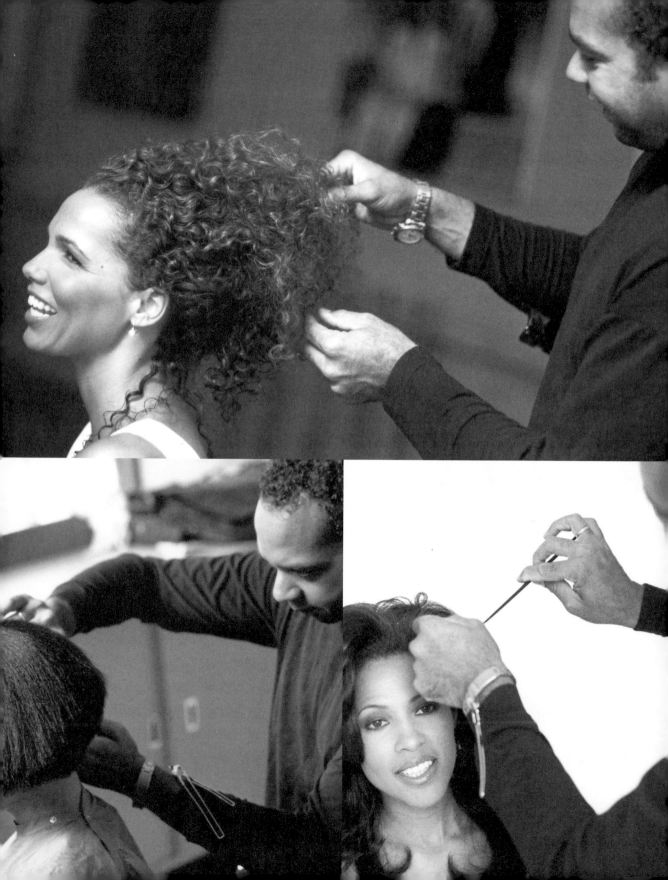

matchmaker, matchmaker

finding the perfect hairstylist for you

Believe it or not, I, too, was once a hair victim. Years ago—more than I care to admit—I was an usher for a major-event company in Chicago. I was a high school student, and it was a great way for me to make some extra cash. At the time—some of you may remember those days—big, fluffy Afros were all the rage. Of course, I had to have one, so I had grown a huge, floppy 'fro that grazed my shoulders and got in my eyes. I loved it. What can I say? It *was* the seventies. But there was just one thing holding me back from total hair bliss: my part-time job required that all ushers wear military-style haircuts. Which meant that my 'fro had to go.

Because I wasn't so willing to give up my crowning glory, I resorted to subterfuge. I rushed out to the drugstore and bought one of those super Afro blowout kits that I'd seen advertised on television. Why? With a logic reserved only for adolescents, I figured that if I blew out my Afro, it would be more manageable and I could slick it back; if I could get it to lay down, no one would notice how long my hair was. No way was I going to succumb to the scissors. So with the help of a friend, I blew out my hair. Except that those blowout kits were nothing more than glorified relaxers. The result? My big, fluffy 'fro was transformed into a limp, lackluster bob that hung lankily over my shoulders. Instead of disguising my long locks, I only managed to make them more noticeable.

Still, I went to work, crossing my fingers, hoping against all hope that my boss wouldn't notice. No such luck. He noticed—and I was promptly sent home. The next day, I was issued an ultimatum: cut your hair or quit. Being the rebellious type, I quit. I still refused to cut my hair. Which was crazy, since I couldn't do anything with this scraggly bob I was now sporting. After a few days of picking it, teasing it, doing anything I could to get it to stand up, I ended up cutting it off anyway. I had no hair and no job.

The moral of this story? Always consult a professional before doing anything drastic to your hair. Had I bothered to talk to a barber or a hairstylist, he would have told me that blowout kits were designed to relax Type 4 hair to more closely resemble Type 3 hair. Since I was already a Type 3, there was no way a blowout kit would give me the look I wanted. I'd still have my hair—and maybe even my job.

The other moral to this story is don't believe the hype. If the label on a hair-color package says "copper-penny red," it doesn't necessarily mean that your hair is going to turn out the color of a penny. "Volume-enhancing" shampoos aren't going to puff up your hair; blowout kits and the like can be a recipe for hair disaster.

By now, you know that I believe strongly that you should leave the big hair jobs to the pros. But that doesn't mean blindly turning your locks over to just any old hairstylist. Now that I've armed you with my tricks of the trade, you're well equipped to be a discerning hair consumer. It's time for you to take all that information out into the world and find the perfect hairstylist for you.

Don't get me wrong: this can be a trial-and-error process. You're not going to click with every stylist, no matter what the buzz surrounding him, no matter how many society divas line up for the chance to sit in her chair. If you and your stylist don't see eye to eye, it doesn't matter if *Vogue* thinks he's the second coming.

So how do you find this perfect person? Ask around. Now that you know your hair type—and how to identify it in others—don't hesitate to stop and ask other women on the street whose hair you admire. It's actually the best way to find someone. Don't rely on photographs in magazines; frequently I find that women who bring in photographs from magazines are really more interested in looking like the model than in her hair.

Take Karen. As a teenager, she would spend hours staring at photos of models in the magazines. Dutifully, she'd cut out the photos and present them to a new stylist in a new salon. She might show them a picture of the figure skater Dorothy Hamill or of Farrah Fawcett or whoever was the "it" model of the minute. But the request was always the same: make me look like that. Invariably, she would be disappointed; somehow, her Type 1 hair would never look like the model's in the photograph, and she'd end up with hair she could do nothing with. No one ever told her, "Your hair is nothing like the model's in the photograph. It's not going to work. Let's try something else." They just took the picture—and her money. So after countless bad haircuts and even worse perms, Karen says she has learned her lesson. She asks around for recommendations. She finds out how long a particular stylist has been in business. She relies on her intuition when she meets a stylist; if it's someone she feels comfortable with and who gives her a great haircut, she's going to come back. When she finds someone good, she sticks with him

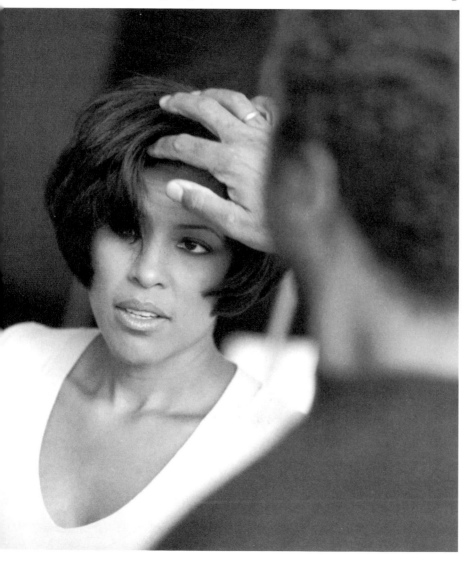

or her for years.

Most of my clients come to me by word of mouth. I cut so-and-so's hair; her girlfriend loved it and wanted to know who did it. So next thing you know, the girlfriend is sitting in my chair. Her buddy loves what I did for her, so she ends up coming to me, too. Or you can pick a salon based on its reputation and ask them to recommend someone who works well with your particular type.

This is an important point: figure out what you want your stylist for. Some stylists are more interested in doing certain types of hair than other types. She might be a curly hair expert; he might love playing with long hair, piling it into elaborate up-'dos. She might be an ace at coloring and highlighting; he might be a whiz at easing kinks into smooth waves. Ask around, tell the stylist what you want. Maybe he or she can cut hair like a dream but doesn't feel comfortable with permanent waves. If my client wants me to do something that I think another stylist in my salon does better, I won't hesitate to tell her. This way, everyone's happy.

Here are what I call the "Top Six Signs That You Should Take Your Money and Run Before Handing Your Hair over to the Hairdresser from Hell":

1. The stylist is lounging around, reading a magazine. Obviously no one else wants him to do their hair.

2. Her hair looks bad. She doesn't care enough to keep her hair in good shape—why would she care about yours?

3. She's wearing a haircut that looks really dated—like Farrah Fawcett's wings. She's stuck in the past, and when she gets done with it, your hair will be, too.

4. He's got you under a faucet, dumping shampoo on your head the minute you walk in the door. If he doesn't bother to take a look at you and ask you about your likes and dislikes, how could he possibly give you a cut that will fit your lifestyle and your type?

5. She's standing over you, scissors in hand, breaking out in a sweat and visibly shaking in her boots. Look out.

6. He comes in with a black eye and spends the rest of the time whining about how he got into a fistfight the night before. If you become friends over the years, that's one thing. But a stylist who can't keep his personal life at home has no business with his hands in your hair. It's just not professional.

The point is, finding a good hairstylist is a business proposition. You're handing over your hard-earned cash; you have every right to expect good service in return. Just be smart and do your homework in advance. Basically, you want a stylist who is busy but available to you. A stylist who is hanging around, gossiping and watching soaps obviously doesn't have enough to do. He's not in demand for a reason. Don't sacrifice your hair trying to find out why. Call ahead, find out if you can come in for a consultation; salons never charge for scheduling chat time with a prospective client. On your first visit, a good hairdresser will examine your hair type, asking you questions about your lifestyle and what you've been doing to your hair. She'll go through a list of chemicals, and ask you if you've used any of them. He'll want to know how much time you're willing to spend on your hair.

Your job during this process is to be as honest as possible. If you've committed hair sins like combining permanent color and relaxers, 'fess up. Let the stylist know everything you've done to your hair, chemicalwise, for the last two years. I've had people come to me and tell me that they haven't had any color on their hair in a couple of years. But the reality is, they'd bleached their hair, got tired of it and six months ago dyed it back to its natural color—conveniently forgetting that under that chestnut brown is a platinum-blonde shade, just waiting to grow out. As you know by now, once your hair is chemically treated, it's chemically treated until it grows out or you cut it off.

Remember, your stylist is only human. Don't come in name-dropping about that famous hairstylist on the infomercials who cut your hair five years ago. Intimidating a stylist, especially one relatively new to the business, will only make him or her nervous. Do you want a nervous stylist cutting your hair? Name-dropping can be a total tool of intimidation. I've seen stylists do a great job in the face of blatant name-dropping or crumble under the pressure. It happened to me when I was starting out. A new client would plop down in my chair and "casually" mention that the most famous stylist in town was her regular hairdresser. It cowed me. I would think, "So-and-so is the best there is. I have to compete with that?" Over the years I've learned that, well, so-and-so might have done your hair, but obviously something didn't work out, because you wouldn't be sitting in my chair now. Still, there's never a need to start out in such an adversarial way. If you two click, you'll be seeing a lot of each other over the next few years. Which leads me to another point . . .

breaking up is hard to do

a few years back, when I still owned my own salon, I had a high-profile client who came to me regularly—I'd do her hair twice a week without fail. It was a professional relationship free of complications: I enjoyed doing her hair; she enjoyed having me do her hair. This was the case until the day I was forced to fire one of my stylists—let's call him Alex—for a variety of reasons. Now this client, let's call her Charlene, just *loved* to gossip. She absolutely had to know why Alex "quit." I certainly wasn't talking. So she made an appointment with him at his new job just so she could dig up the dirt. But as they say, God don't like ugly.

One day she was sitting in Alex's chair at his new salon, hair dripping wet, when Donald, one of my stylists, dropped by to visit Alex. Of course it got back to me that Charlene was two-timing me with Alex. She was so embarrassed that she never came back to my salon. She didn't show up for her appointments; she wouldn't return my phone calls. It was too awkward for her to come back. To this day, she has never come clean with me—not even when she appeared on Oprah's show and I did her hair. She never talked about what happened, and I never brought it up.

The moral of this story? Breaking up with your hairstylist is hard to do. It seems silly, but if you've been with your stylist for years, deciding to move on can create a sticky situation. You've developed a relationship built on trust. He has seen you at your absolute worst and has helped you to look your absolute best. She's talked you out of cutting your hair off immediately after you dumped your last significant

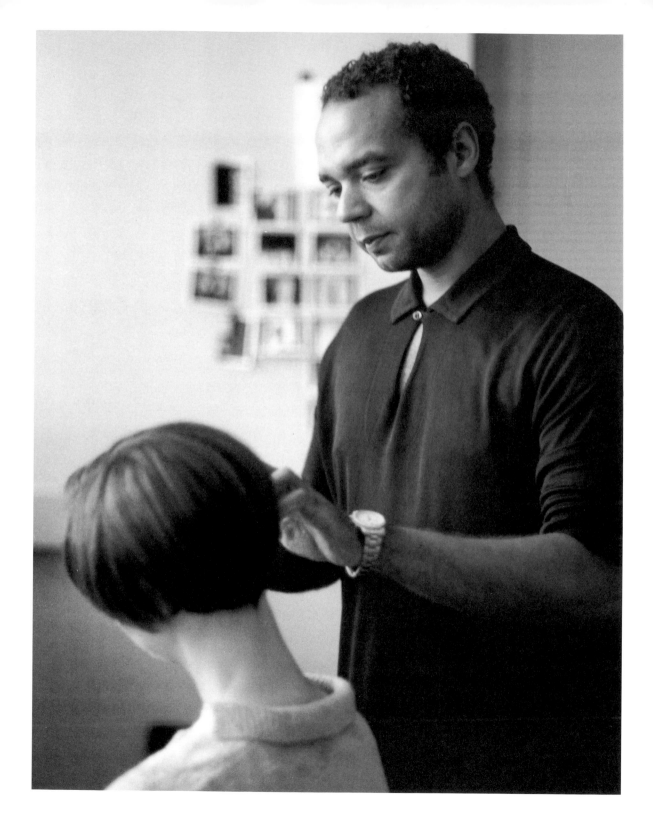

other. He's helped you through some serious hair uglies, including the time when your hair was shedding faster than a molting snake and you were convinced that you'd be wearing wigs for the rest of your life. But suddenly you just don't jibe anymore. She keeps cutting your hair off when you insist that, this time, you want to let it grow. Or he just doesn't seem interested in you as a client anymore, keeping you waiting for hours while he squeezes in some socialite ahead of you. Going to the salon shouldn't be a tortuous experience. So, as in any relationship, when you're unhappy more often than you're happy, it's time to go.

But while most women's magazines run regular articles on how to dump an unworthy lover, there's no advice out there on how to break up with your stylist. There's no protocol to follow, no set guidelines written up in the hairdresser's bible. Still, there are things you can do to ease the transition. Don't be a chicken like my friend Terry and simply stop going. Now, every time she spies her ex—stylist, that is—she crosses the street to avoid her. Do tell your stylist that you're not happy; tell her that you want to try someone new. This is an especially important step if you want to try someone else in the same salon. Most stylists, while they won't enjoy hearing this, will be gracious. It happens to the best of us; it's happened to me, too. But at this point in my career, it doesn't bother me as much. I know that if I lose a client, it's not going to kill me or my business. I try to look at it logically. Maybe this person doesn't like the way that I do hair; maybe she'll find someone whose work she does like. It doesn't mean that I'm not a good stylist; it just means that we're not a good fit. So whatever you do, don't stick with someone who doesn't make you happy.

on the other hand . . . finding an alternative

maybe you're thrilled with your hairdresser. She's just . . . busy. If your stylist is any good, there are going to be times when he's just not available. Maybe she's doing photo shoots for a magazine. Maybe he's doing hair on a movie location. Maybe she's just booked for the next three months, and you need to see someone right away. Don't get left in the lurch: make sure that you have option number two waiting in the wings. I'm not talking mutiny here. Of course, you're going to have that one hairdresser to whom you're most loyal, but it's always good to have a second choice whom you can rely on in a pinch. My mom and sister will go to other people when I'm not in town. I tell all my clients that they should do the same. I'm often out of town for months at a stretch; during this time, my clients need to know that there's someone else who can handle their hair. I tell them to be up front with their second choice. You should be, too.

Tell the stylist, "Listen, I have a stylist that I normally go to. I'm very happy with him, but he's not available right now and I hear that you're very good. I'm going to use you as my alternative." If you find that they give you a great hairstyle but are always trying to steal you away as a regular client, forget it. Most mature stylists are comfortable with being the hairdresser on the side; most are happy just to have the business. They're happy that someone thought enough of their work to recommend their services. If a client goes to someone else while I'm away and comes back with a new suggestion from the other stylist, if it's legitimate, I'll consider it. Why not? Your relationship with your stylist *should* be an open marriage. So don't be afraid to ask your regular stylist for a recommendation.

one more thing

know that these days money is tight. You've got to feed the credit card beast. Maybe you've got student loans to pay off, or maybe the kids are in college. Maybe you're living on a fixed income; maybe you're a single mom struggling to pay the bills. Whichever the case may be, cash is tight. I've been there, and I know it's not easy. Still, you should resist the urge to skimp on your hair.

I'm not fond of haircutting chains, because there's no quality control. Yes, they're dirt cheap—who can beat an eight-dollar haircut? The only problem is, you usually end up looking like you have an eight-dollar haircut—or worse. Yes, there are good hairstylists working at these chains. The problem is, there's no guarantee that you're going to get one on a regular basis. Chains operate on a drop-in basis: whoever's available is who you're going to get. Even if you've got the simplest of bobs, it's still important to have hair that's cut well.

So what do you do if you can't afford to go to an expensive salon? Figure out what your budget can accommodate comfortably, then shop around for a quality salon that meets your budget requirements. Get a cut that doesn't require a lot of upkeep, something like a shoulder-length bob that's easy and neat and only requires reshaping every other month or so. Resist the urge to experiment with costly and time-consuming chemical procedures. Keep it simple.

Still, you should consider your hair an investment. Finding a good stylist should be a priority. Look for someone who cares about how well he or she does your hair and how well it looks. Like it or not, this society still judges people based on how they look, so your appearance is very important. Plus, you'll feel much better about yourself when you're looking your absolute best. And isn't that what life is all about?

I went into this business to make people happy. I truly believe that when you look good, you feel good—and vice versa. A friend once told me that she thought my purpose in life was not just to make people look better, but to make them feel better about themselves. I'd like to think that I've accomplished that in some way during my twenty-year career, which is why I wrote this book. If in these pages I've given you some information you can actually use *and* have helped you to feel just a little bit better about yourself and the beauty God handed you, then I'm a happy man.

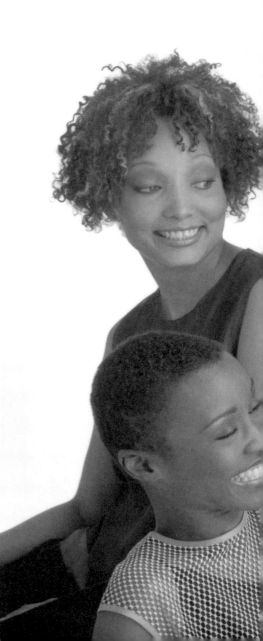

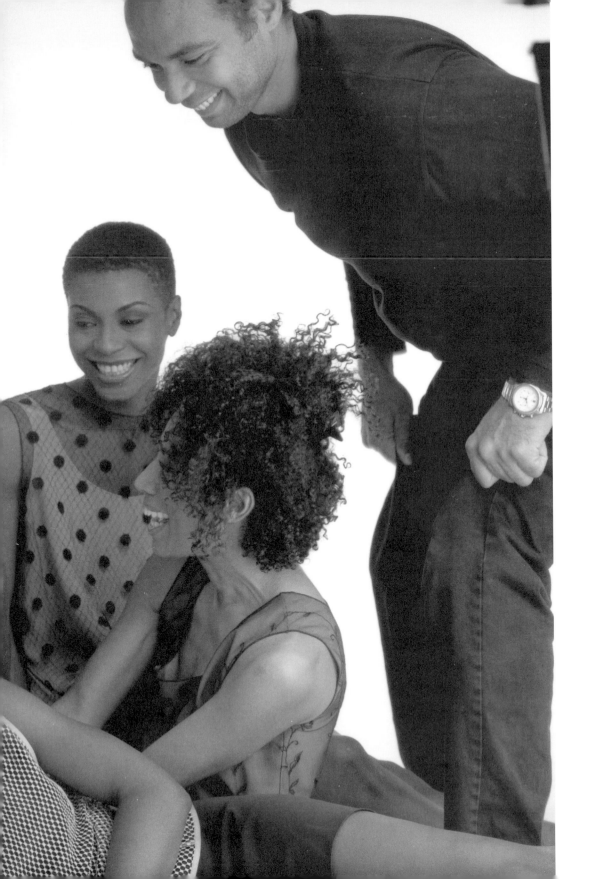

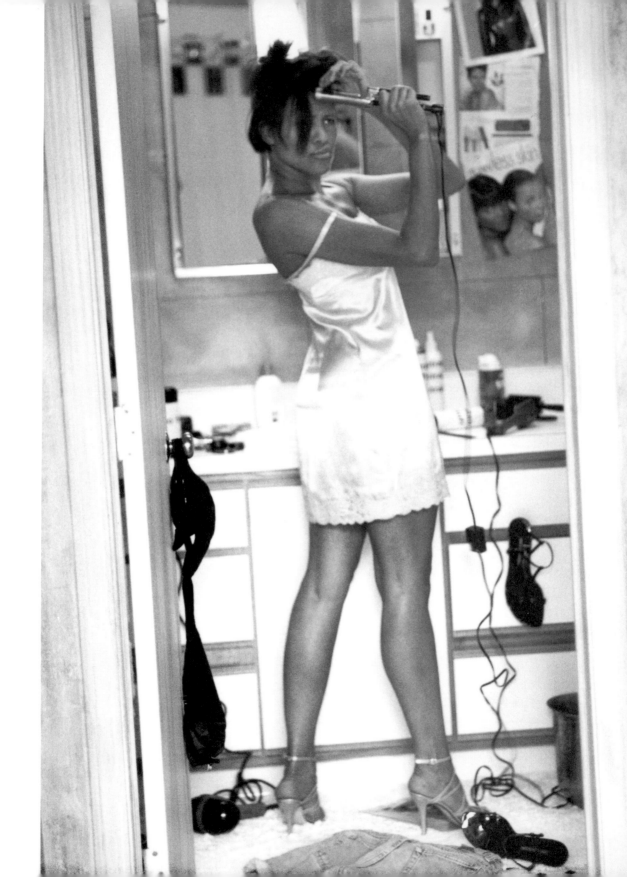

doing the 'do

taking matters into your own hands

Nobody, but nobody, beats Madonna when it comes to quick-change hairdos—not even Patti LaBelle with her outrageous stage 'dos. One minute Madonna is Marilyn Monroe, the next she's sporting brunette waves; she's doing a mod shag, then she's looking very retro with her bleached *Evita* twists and chignons. Her hairdos show true creative genius—someone else's creative genius. All you have to do is take one look at her elaborately presented coifs to know that somewhere, waiting in the wings, there's a nimble-fingered professional hairstylist armed with a comb, brush, hairpins and hairspray. But most of us don't have it like that, let's face it—very few of us can afford to have a hairstylist following us around at all times. Still, you don't have to have me on retainer or even be especially talented with a comb and brush to achieve a variety of looks. All you need are a few simple tools (more on that later), a little know-how and a little encouragement to look fabulously different within minutes.

Encouragement is the key word here. Variety is the spice of life, but many women cling to that one tried-and-true 'do because they're insecure about their looks. Once they think they've found that one magic style that suits them, they're afraid to venture into uncharted territory. A big reason for this is that they've internalized ridiculous things that people have told them over the years; it takes a lot of courage to ignore those old voices. One client, let's call her Kerri, was told as a tenth grader that she looked sick whenever she pulled her hair back. Today she's in her thirties, and she still worries that she looks tired or worn out whenever she heads out the door with her security blanket pinned up, even though I think that she looks great with a sleek chignon. She thinks of it as a bad hair day 'do—a mistaken notion to which a lot of women subscribe. Up-'dos, ponytails, French twists, buns, etc., etc., are seen as a last resort—reserved for those days when you can't do a thing with your hair. This is a shame, because those 'dos needn't be hair-styling stepchildren. They are legitimate—not to mention chic—in their own right.

Then there are women like Oprah, who never want to be seen without a fringe of bangs covering their forehead. They think their forehead is too big, or too wide, or too small, or too narrow, or just too too. It doesn't matter that they have a really nice face; they don't see it that way. Trying to get those clients to confront the world with a face unconcealed by hair is a major undertaking. Sometimes, to shake things up a bit, I'll just go ahead and style Oprah's hair without bangs. I generally don't like to do that, but sometimes you have to take a risk to encourage someone to change. It's hard to step out of your mold without the reassurance that you really do look nice. Once you summon the courage to try something new, and others compliment you, then it's that much easier the next time. It's the proverbial catch-22: you can't get the positive reassurance you need to make a change until you take a deep breath and go for it.

Of course, some women are chameleons by nature. They thrive on change and feel comfortable sporting a number of different looks. I love change; still, a few guidelines are in order. Namely, don't go overboard. A little restraint is essential! Don't make the mistake of going for all-out glamour with an overdone 'do; don't tease your bangs so that they enter the room before you do and then forget about the rest of your hair. You want to look tempting, not tacky. I'm talking about indulging in a few simple changes—pinning your hair up in an easy French twist. Curling it one day instead of wearing it straight. Slicking short hair back with gel for a wet look. Small changes can have a big impact. To achieve this, all you'll need are a few basic tools (which ones depend on your hair type and length): a curling iron, comb, brush, hairpins that match your hair color, styling combs, butterfly clamps, covered ponytail holders, a large hairclip and gel. Are you ready? Let's get busy.

a quick diversion with braids

Some days, your ultra-long dreads or braids can make you feel like you're holding the weight of the world on your shoulders. Take a load off with this quick-change up-'do.

Tools
• Hairpins that match the color of your braids

Steps
• Throw head forward and gather braids up into a top ponytail.
• Take a few braids from each side of the front part of hair.
• Crisscross braids in front of ponytail, wrap around toward back of ponytail and secure at base with a couple of hairpins.

Tips
• Don't make the ponytail too tight because you can put too much stress on your natural hair (you can also pull your braids out).
• Use a light conditioning oil or braid sheen on your braids to keep them looking healthy and shiny.

braids

sleek and shiny

sleek and shiny

W ant a new look for that short cut? You can achieve some of the best looks with gel. That slicked back Josephine Baker look will be an easy distraction from that everyday bob. With this 'do, you might just feel like doing the hoochy-coo topless and in a banana.

Tools
- Fine-tooth comb
- Brush
- Gel

Steps
- Wash hair and towel dry.
- Apply gel and work through hair with a fine-tooth comb.
- Comb into desired shape and let set until dry.
- For a softer look, run a brush through hair after it is completely dry.

Tip
• For the best results, look for a non-flaking gel.

the undone up-'do

You've got "day-old" hair that's got to look brand new—and you've got ten minutes to shower, dress and feed your rottweiler before your date starts pounding on your door. Grab some hairpins. Help is on the way . . .

Tools

• Brush

• Hairpins the color of your hair

• Decorative combs or chopsticks (if desired)

Steps

• Gently brush hair back and gather toward the nape of your neck.

• Twist hair upward toward the crown and secure with hairpins.

• Leaving the ends untucked, style loosely by pulling small wispy sections of your hair down to softly frame your face.

Tip

• For something different, secure twist with decorative chopsticks or combs.

the undone up-'do

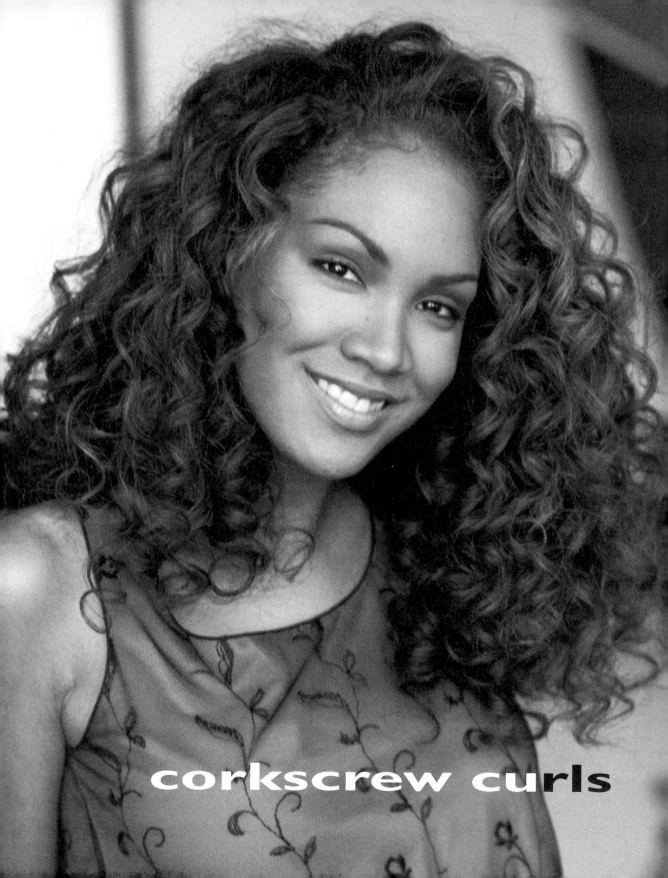

corkscrew curls

corkscrew curls

So you look like Cher but yearn for Nicole Kidman's pre-Raphaelite curls. Before you reach for the Toni's Home Permanent solution, try my not-so-permanent alternative.

Tools
• Curling iron
• Large hairclip

Steps
• Separate a small section of hair and clip the rest.
• Loosely twist the small section of hair.
• While holding an open curling iron, wrap the twisted section of hair around the barrel from the base of the hair to the end in a spiral motion and close the iron for a few seconds.
• When the curl is set, slide curling iron out.
• Do not break up the curl by combing—just style with fingers.

Tip
• For tighter curls, spray each section before curling with a light holding spray and use a smaller curling iron.

crown of curls

the heat is on, and your long, curly locks are starting to make you feel like it's way above 100° outside. It's summertime, and this hairdo is easy . . .

Tools

• Brush

• Ponytail holder

• Bobby pins that match the color of your hair

Steps

• Pull the front and sides of your hair up into a ponytail.

• Continue gathering sections in an upward sweep, adding to your ponytail until all of your hair is piled up.

• Secure.

Tip

• For those of you with thick tresses, or if you're looking for a looser cascade of curls, try this method:

1. Attach a long or medium-length bobby pin to each end of a ponytail holder.

2. Gather your hair in a ponytail in one hand.

3. Secure one bobby pin at the base of the ponytail.

4. Wrap the ponytail holder around the base of the ponytail at least once, and secure the other bobby pin on the opposite side.

crown of curls

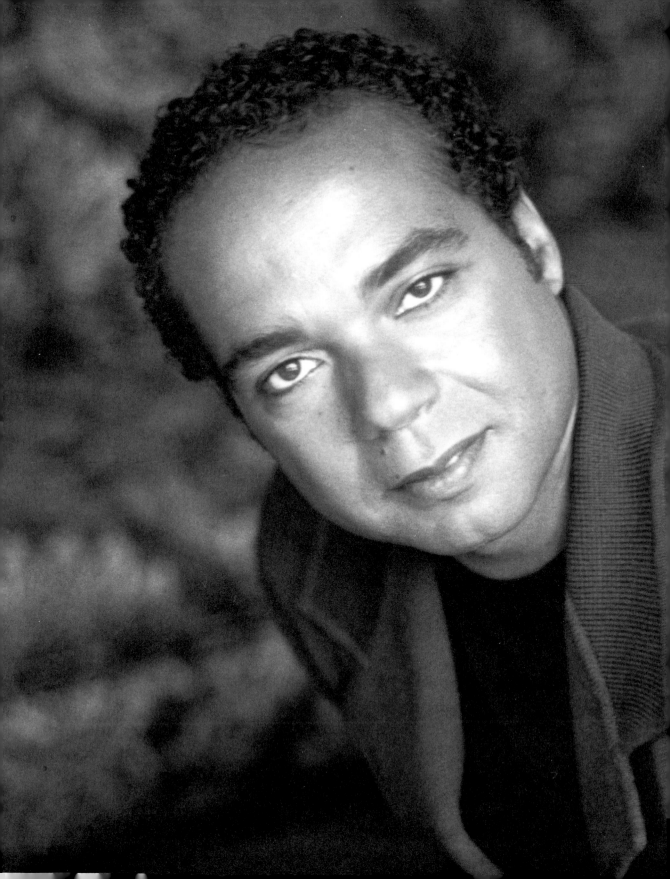

ask andre

answers to your most common hairstyling questions

Q I've lost weight; I'm eating right. But I can't do anything with my Type 4 hair. I'm losing my hair and I'm not sure why. I have gone to several doctors, and no one seems to be able to find the problem. I would love advice on what to do. I have spent thousands of dollars on doctors; I'm willing to spend thousands more to find the answer. I'm working out a lot, trying to keep my dress size down, but it doesn't help my hair. Please help me.

A My guess is that you're not losing your hair; it's simply breaking off. If you have Type 4 hair that you relax, you might get some breakage when you start to work out if you don't get regular touch-ups. This happens when your hair starts to grow out; the hair at your roots is much more tightly curled than the rest of your processed hair. When you work out, the moisture from the perspiration on your scalp makes the new growth kink up while the rest of your hair remains straight. When you comb your hair after a workout, the comb snags over the two radically different textures. The result? Hair that snaps off in your comb. Instant free haircut. To remedy this, you can do one of two things. Get regular touch-ups every four to six weeks so that your hair is straight, and shampoo and style your hair following each and every workout. Or opt for a short, natural cut that works beautifully with the kinks and curls of your Type 4 hair. With either method, you should see a vast improvement in your hair condition. Of course, it goes without saying that if your hair is actually falling out, and you can see smooth, shiny bald patches, you should see a doctor immediately.

Q I just finished working out and I am in tears. My hair looks crazy. I am on the verge of quitting. I don't know if the workout is worth my feeling bad about the way my hair looks. I have even cut down on the intensity of my workouts because of the hair issue. The ultimate would be to work out as hard as I could every day and not worry about my hair. Do you have any suggestions?

A Whatever type hair you have, if you exercise frequently, I suggest that you stick with your natural hair texture. Find a style that you can just wash and wear, a 'do that requires no more upkeep than a dollop of gel before you head out the door. There are styles in every single hair texture that will allow you to do just that. You have to decide if you want a highly coiffed hairstyle every day, or if you want to work out hard every day and sport a simple, flattering haircut. Don't abandon your workouts because of your hair. Keep exercising. You want more than just your hair to look good.

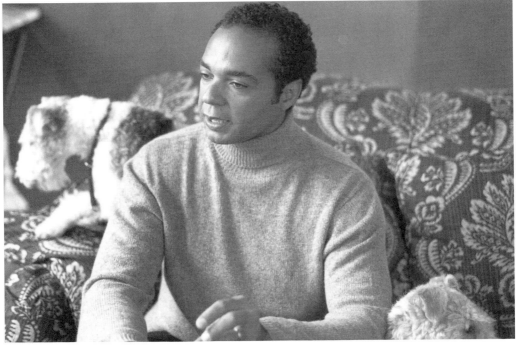

Q My daughter needs your help. It's not life or death, but to a fourteen-year-old, it's pretty important. The problem is her hair! I'm white and her father is black. My daughter has a blond Afro. It is so thick, dry, frizzy, poofy, etc. She almost always wears it in ponytails. She is a very pretty girl, but I wish I could do something with her Afro! We have gone to expensive salons, white beauticians, black beauticians. We've used straighteners, hair food, conditioners, you name it, we've probably tried it. There are many beautiful black women with straight hair, and I just don't know how they do it and if it could be done to my daughter.

A A blond Afro can be very beautiful. Chrystelle, a black French supermodel, made a name for herself on the runway with her distinct looks and big, fluffy, sandy-blond Afro. Straight or straightened hair does not make someone beautiful. If it's really important for your daughter to have relaxed hair, she's old enough to learn how to maintain that style—if that's what she wants. Look for a good hairstylist in your area who's willing to teach her how to maintain relaxed hair. But most of all, your daughter needs to learn to work with her natural hair texture and appreciate its own unique beauty. If she wants to wear her hair natural, help her find a nice, cute hairstyle that will flatter her hair. Read Chapter 3, "Care and Feeding," for tips on caring for Type 3 or Type 4 hair. But most of all, tell your daughter that you think she and her hair are beautiful as they are.

Q I've been a stylist for over twenty years and have a little trouble with chemical straightening. I am assuming that Oprah has some sort of chemical relaxing done, and yet her hair looks perfectly healthy. Please share your secret. I have a few frizzy-haired clients who are in desperate need!

A Frizzy hair doesn't mean that you need to run for the nearest jar of chemical relaxer. Frizzy hair actually comes in several hair types. Your clients could have very coarse, wavy Type 2 hair that frizzes. Putting a chemical relaxer on that type of hair would be a mistake. Instead, it can be smoothed out with a blow-dryer. Relaxers wouldn't take the frizz out of that particular hair type, whereas other frizzy types might benefit from the judicious use of a chemical straightener. As with all chemical processes, you can count on the hair drying out to a certain degree. It's important to make sure that chemically treated hair is conditioned and moisturized following each shampoo. I cannot stress that enough. Read Chapter 5, "Messing with Mother Nature," for more on caring for relaxed hair.

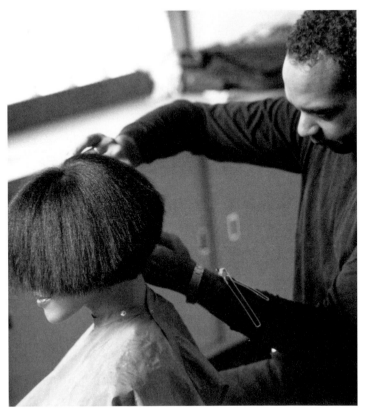

Q I want to change my style, but to what? I'm always open to change; I get bored with the same look. But what look is right? How do the professionals judge? Do you judge the shape of the face or do you take body type and size into account as well? Would someone who is plump wear short, cropped hair? Is it better to keep a certain length? Questions, questions.

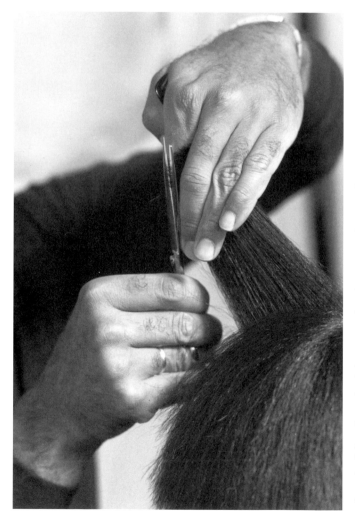

A I don't believe that there is any set formula. Yes, you do take face shape and body size into account, but there aren't any rules in the beauty game. It's not necessarily true that large-sized women can't wear short hair. You have to decide if a particular style works for your hair texture— not to mention the rest of you. It's a trial-and-error thing. Don't be afraid to experiment. And when you're done, ask a friend for her honest (and tactful) opinion.

Q How do you style hair that continually falls out? I'm too scared to brush it, let alone style it. Help!

A Your hair could be falling out for a number of reasons. Before you figure out which hairstyle will best disguise your problem, figure out what's *causing* the problem. See a hairstylist first. If he or she can't help you, then you need to see a dermatologist. Your problem could be medical, or it could be something very simple. I once had a client whose hair was falling out in clumps. It turned out that she'd been highlighting her naturally dark hair; the highlighted hair was falling out from chemical damage. That was a problem I could easily solve as a hairstylist. I simply told her to stop bleaching her highlights and opt instead for not-so-blond highlights.

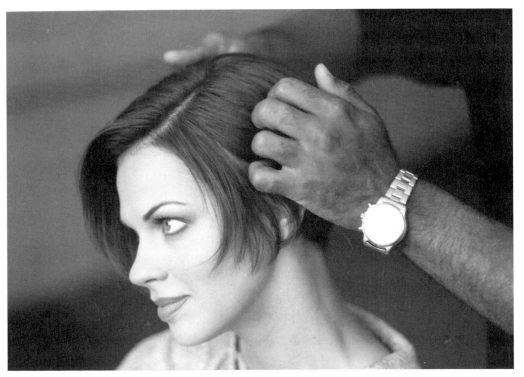

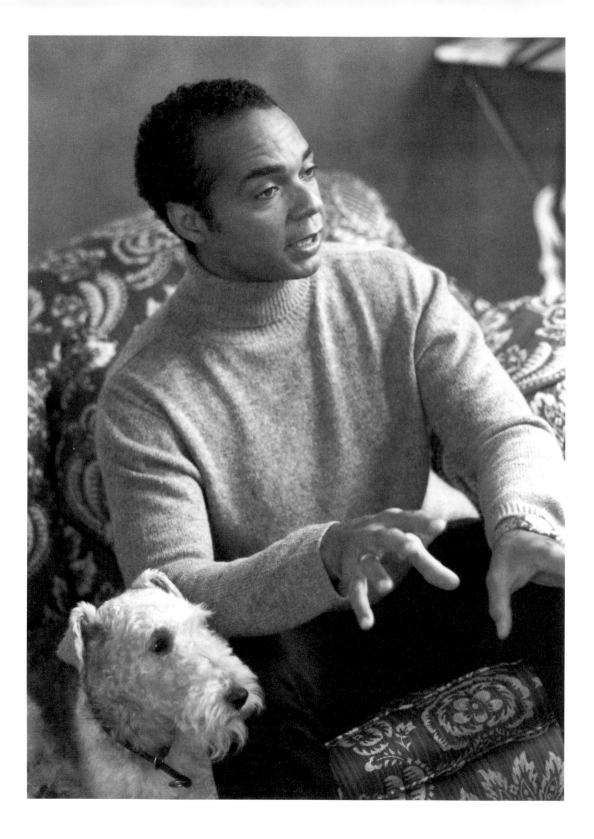

Q I just had my first child a year ago. Before the birth of my son, I had wonderful naturally curly, thick hair. Now, I still have the thickness but my hair has lost its curl. I don't even know where to begin with hairstyles. I don't know how to manage straight hair. I am desperate and don't know what to do.

A It's not unusual for your hair texture to change following the birth of a baby. More than likely, your hair will return to its natural texture at some point; your texture won't be changed permanently. But with the hormonal changes still raging in your body, it might take awhile. In the meantime, find a style that works well with straight hair; don't fight your current texture. Get your hairdresser to teach you how to take care of your "new" hair. Make what you have right now work for you.

Q I lost 75 percent of my hair after going through four surgeries within a twelve-month period. I've tried everything—even rinsing it with warm apple cider vinegar as a friend suggested. It's just smelly, not helpful.

A Your body has been through a lot in the past year; surgery is a traumatic experience. While losing that much hair can be frightening, it's not unexpected after all you've been through. Don't panic. If you haven't already, see a dermatologist to find out what you can do; this isn't a task for a stylist. You might have to play the waiting game. Your hair might not grow back until you're completely healthy. In the meantime, read Chapter 7, "Damage Control." Invest in some attractive scarves, hats and wigs. And put away the vinegar. Homemade recipes rarely work in these instances.

Q I love my hairdresser (would move if she did), but I would love a change. My gray is covered by a blend of five different shades. I would love to try a different shade, but I'm scared. What do you suggest for someone whose idea of "doing my hair" means washing it in the shower and using a blow-dryer and my fingers to style it?

A You don't have to leave your hairdresser to change your hair color. If you don't live in a major city, take a trip to the city nearest you and look up a salon that specializes in hair color, one known for doing beautiful color. You can find such a salon by reading fashion magazines that do roundups listing the best salons in the country. Once you find your salon, go in for a free consultation before you invest in your new color. Tell the stylist that you want a new look. Later, your regular stylist can help you maintain your new color. Change is a good thing. Sometimes one good hairdresser can learn from and appreciate what another good hairdresser has to offer. So don't worry about offending your tried-and-true stylist.

Q I have very fine, thin blond hair. I want to add just a little more body to my hair. I do not want any more perms! My hairdresser has suggested applying the hair-color product Shades to my hair. Do you think this will help?

A Applying temporary colors like Shades would help. It will give your hair a little more body, but not much. It will just coat the hair, making it appear a little fuller than it is. Permanent color like highlights, lowlights, anything using peroxide will expand the cuticle of the hair, making it fuller from the chemical process.

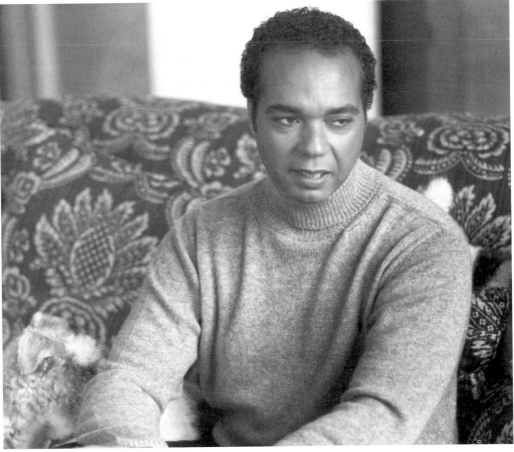

Q How can I find a good "curly hair" hairdresser?

A Look for women on the street who have your hair type (and look good) and ask them, "Where did you get your hair done?" That's always the best way to find out.

Q My beautiful mom is seventy-four years old and is allergic to peroxide and other things in hair color. However, she can use some of the temporary rinses to cover her gray. But sometimes they turn a greenish color, and right now she has some interesting shades of red and pink in her hair. Please, please tell me how to start from scratch and make corrections. She is really shy about going to a hairdresser because when she was sixty-eight she had an aneurysm and has had several surgeries that have left large indentations and scars on her head. I'd love to help her feel better about her hair.

A Take your mom to a hair-color specialist. Get someone to take patch tests on your mom to see which hair-color products cause an allergic reaction. With a patch test, the colorist will test different chemicals by dabbing a small sample on the client's arm. If all is well after twenty-four hours, then it's safe to proceed with the hair color. One is bound to work for your mom. But please, leave the coloring to the hair-color experts. A well-trained professional won't give your mom pink hair and will be sensitive about her surgical scars.

Q I am Caucasian, with very curly hair. Not like African-American hair, but very curly. Since I was a little girl, I've been trying to figure out what to do with it. One time I was so frustrated that I cut it so short that I couldn't even grab it. When it's wet, it looks great; it doesn't look so great when it's dry. I can't brush it because that makes it look very kinky. Right now, I'm wearing it shoulder length, but I always have it tied in a bun or a braid because I don't have a good cut. I have been cutting it myself for over five years. I would love to find a "curly hair salon." I don't want to have to blow-dry it straight or do anything that takes too long to style. I am a very busy professional woman and single mom.

A Your first mistake was in cutting your own hair. Don't do it! It's very difficult to cut your own hair and make it look good. A professional who is used to cutting curly hair is the only person you should trust with your hair. Invest in a good haircut first. Ask around; find other women with good-looking curly hair and ask them to point you to their stylist. You might want to check out salons that specialize in African-American or very curly hair. Very curly, textured Type 3 or Type 4 hair comes in all ethnicities. Even if you have to travel to find a good stylist, do it. You're worth it. Then experiment with different styling products that will help control your hair. On "good hair days," analyze what you did differently, then try to duplicate that every day.

acknowledgments

If I'd tried to do this on my own, this book would have remained nothing more than an idea. So there are a few folks out there to whom I owe major thanks.

Thanks to God for making all of this happen.

My family, especially my mother and sister Pam, for being guinea pigs way back when, when my hair obsession first began. Thanks for always being there for me.

A special thanks to Oprah, for her guidance and friendship—and for giving me a chance way back when.

Harpo Studios, for the use of their studio during the photo shoots for this book. Thanks to everyone there for making this task much, much easier.

David, for his unending support.

My good friend Howell A. Johnson for all of his advice, support and extraordinary ideas.

Shirley and Lucas for all their kisses.

All my loyal clients who were so generous in allowing me to release some of my creative frustration onto their heads.

Jonith Breadon, M.D., for her invaluable expertise in fleshing out Chapter 7.

I want to thank the gang at Simon & Schuster for all their help and effort in putting the book together. First and foremost, my editor Dawn Marie Daniels, I couldn't have done it without you. Carolyn Reidy and Michele Martin for believing in me. Last, but most certainly not least, much thanks to Bonni Leon-Berman, Amy Hill, Theresa Horner, Mary Reed, Jim Thiel, Sam Potts and Melody Guy for making sure everything came out the way we envisioned the book way back when.

I'd also like to thank my agent Denise Stinson.

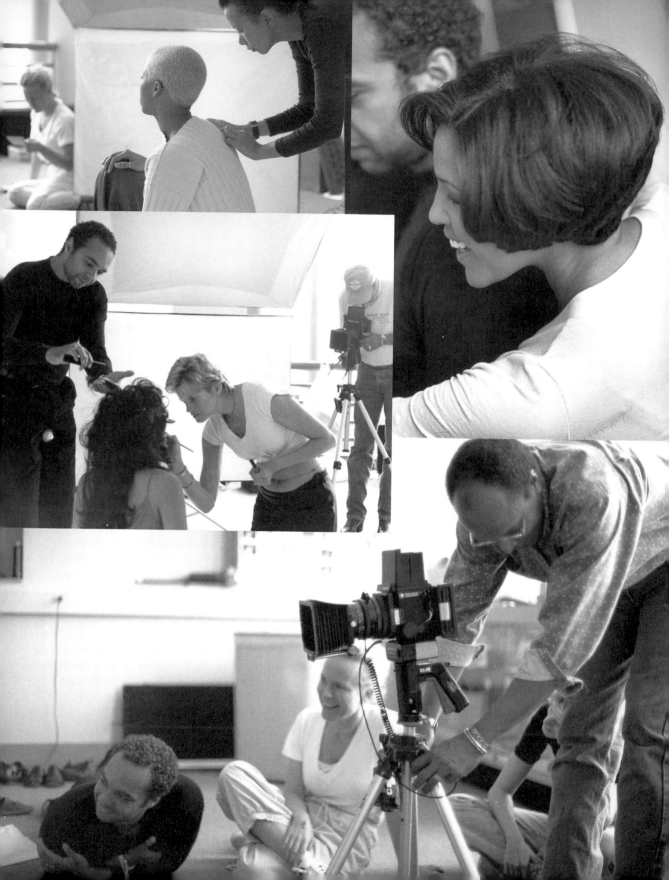

contributors

Teresa Wiltz (writer) is on the staff of the *Chicago Tribune*, where she has covered everything from fashion to crime to the Los Angeles riots to education to arts and entertainment. A graduate of Dartmouth College, Wiltz has written for *Essence* and *Business Week* and was a contributor to the book *Body & Soul: The Black Woman's Guide to Physical Health and Emotional Well-Being*. She lives in Chicago.

Cynthia Moore (creative director/project coordinator), previously a model with Elite Chicago, changed her twelve-year career in front of the camera into one behind the scenes. She put her vast knowledge of and experience in the fashion and beauty industries to use as the fashion editor of a Chicago social magazine for two and a half years. Miss Moore has now focused her Chicago-based career on the production of print, film and books.

John Beckett (photographer) is a twenty-year veteran whose award-winning work has appeared in *Money, Child, Family Circle, Essence, Men's Fitness* and *Inside Sports*. He lives in Scottsdale, Arizona.

Darcy McGrath (makeup artist, photographer, educator) has worked in the fashion and beauty industry for the past seventeen years. Her makeup artistry has appeared in numerous editorial publications including *Vanity Fair* and Italian *Vogue*, and has touched such faces as Jodie Foster, Oprah Winfrey, Andie MacDowell and R.E.M. McGrath creates beauty for all ages and colors, and debuts her eye for photography in Chapter 6. Her private makeup studio is in Chicago.

credits

Creative Director / Project Coordinator	Cynthia Moore
Written by	Teresa Wiltz

Photography

Photographs	John Beckett
Contributing photographs (chapter 6)	Darcy McGrath
Assistant on Camera	Dave Vacula
Photo Assistant	Sam Moon
Photo Assistants (chapter 6)	Michael Pawlowski
	Doug Fogalson

Hair

Direction	Andre Walker
Stylist for Oprah Winfrey	Andre Walker
Hair Colorist	Christopher Bozarth

Contributing Stylists

For the Marianne Strokirk Salon	Osmane Cunha
	Frances Gillespie
	Michael Jacobson
	Anthony Marino
	Lisa Nilson
	Patricia Spata
	Misako Weaver

Makeup

Makeup	Darcy McGrath
Assistant makeup artists	Melanie Randolf
	Tina Turnbow
Makeup for Oprah Winfrey	Fran Cooper
Makeup for *The Oprah Winfrey Show*	Roosevelt Cartwright

Wardrobe

Fashion Stylist	Mia Velez
Assistant Fashion Stylist	Wen Li
Wardrobe	Ultimo, Ltd.
	Jill Sander Chicago
	Giorgio Armani Chicago
	Isacc Mizrahi
	The Wolford Boutique
	SU-ZEN
	Marshall Fields
	Londo Mondo
	Nike

Special Locations

Harpo Studios
Brad's Gym

Cover Credits

Creative Director	Cynthia Moore
Art Director / Designer	Jackie Seow
Photographer	John Beckett
Makeup	Darcy McGrath
Fashion Stylist	Patric Chauvéz
Hair Direction	Andre Walker
Assistant Makeup Artist	Tina Turnbow
Assistant on Camera	Dave Vacula
Assistant Fashion Stylist	Daena Joyce Ogden
Contributing Hairstylists	Osmane Cunha
	Frances Gillespie
	Anthony Marino
	Misako Weaver
Wardrobe	Ultimo Ltd.
Models	Annette Caleel
	Lynn Eggers
	Kelly Mailey
	Eleanor Simon
	Jahaila Sing
	Jennifer Wisniewski

index